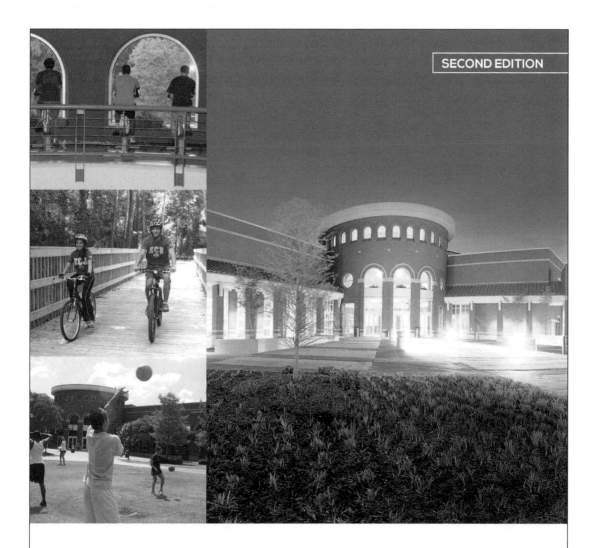

SECOND EDITION

FITNESS MATTERS

LIFETIME PHYSICAL ACTIVITY & FITNESS **LABORATORY MANUAL**

MATTHEW T. MAHAR · THOMAS D. RAEDEKE · MICHAEL R. McCAMMON
C. DAVID KEMBLE · RHONDA K. KENNY · SUSAN L. COHEN

EAST CAROLINA UNIVERSITY

bluedoor
flexible & affordable learning solutions™

Chief Executive Officer: Jon K. Earl

President, College: Lucas Tomasso
President, Private Sector: Dawn Earl

Print Solutions Manager: Connie Dayton
Digital Solutions Manager: Amber Wahl
Content Solutions Manager: Anne Loyle-Langholz
Developmental & Production Coordinator: Meg Olstad
Senior Project Coordinator: Dan Woods
Senior Project Coordinator: Peggy Li
Project Coordinator: Erica Nilsen
Project Coordinator: Kelli Fleck
Project Coordinator: Kristin Bechthold
Production Assistant: Stephanie Larson
Production Assistant: Jessie Steigauf

Cover Design: Dan Woods

ISBN-13: 978-1-68135-228-2

© 2017 by Department of Exercise and Sport Science — East Carolina University and bluedoor, LLC.

© Cover images by Department of Exercise and Sport Science, ECU.

Published by bluedoor, LLC
    10949 Bren Road East
    Minneapolis, MN 55343-9613
    800-979-1624
    www.bluedoorpublishing.com

Printed in the United States of America.
10 9 8 7 6 5 4 3 2 1

TABLE OF CONTENTS

ABOUT THE AUTHORS

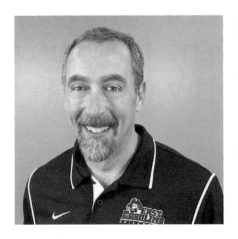

Matt Mahar is a professor in the Department of Kinesiology at East Carolina University and Director of the Activity Promotion Laboratory. He holds a BS degree in Physical Education from SUNY Cortland and an MEd in Exercise Science and an EdD in Measurement and Research in Exercise Science from the University of Houston. Dr. Mahar has taught and coached at the high school level, and has performed research at institutions ranging from the Cardiopulmonary Lab at NASA/Johnson Space Center in Houston, Texas to Pitt County Schools. He is a member of the FitnessGram Scientific Advisory Board and a former member of the President's Council for Fitness, Sports and Nutrition Science Board. Dr. Mahar received the University of North Carolina Board of Governors Award for Excellence in Teaching and the East Carolina University Scholar-Teacher Award.

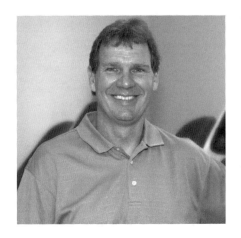

Tom Raedeke is a professor and Graduate Program Director in the Department of Kinesiology at East Carolina University. As a former collegiate wrestler, Dr. Raedeke earned his BA degree from Concordia College in Moorhead, MN, his master's degree from the University of Idaho, and a PhD from the University of Oregon. Dr. Raedeke has taught sport and exercise psychology courses at the University of Oregon, University of Colorado, and East Carolina University. He has received the University of North Carolina Board of Governors Award for Excellence in Teaching, the University of North Carolina Board of Governors Distinguished Professor for Teaching Award, and the East Carolina University Scholar-Teacher Award. He is a certified consultant through the *Association of Applied Sport Psychology* (AASP) where he has served as the chair of the health and exercise psychology focus area. Dr. Raedeke has also served as the chair of the *Sport and Exercise Psychology Academy* and is currently on the executive board for the *North American Society for the Psychology of Sport and Physical Activity*. Prior to university employment, he was a research assistant in coaching education through the American Coaching Effectiveness Program/Human Kinetics Publishing and in sport psychology at the United States Olympic Training Center in Colorado Springs.

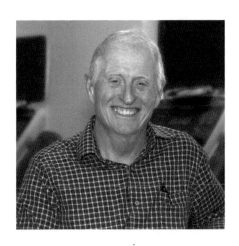

Mike McCammon has been a faculty member at East Carolina University since 1984. He currently serves as the director of the Exercise Physiology BS degree. Mike is a past recipient of the University of North Carolina Board of Governors Distinguished Professor for Teaching Award, ECU advising award, and Scholar-Teacher Award. In his spare time he enjoys walking, very slow jogging, golf, cooking, and kayak fishing.

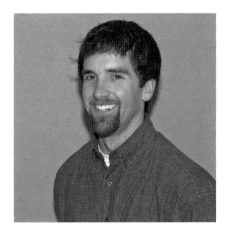

Dave Kemble earned both his BS and MA degrees from East Carolina University. He is an Instructor in the Department of Kinesiology and serves as the Assistant Director of the Activity Promotion Laboratory. Dave is an advisor to undergraduate students in the Health Fitness Specialist degree option where he also teaches courses in Measurement of Physical Activity and Fitness, Personal Fitness Training, and Essentials of Strength and Conditioning. He also serves as the Head Coach for the East Carolina University Olympic Weightlifting Club. Prior to joining the faculty at East Carolina University, Dave worked in the health club industry for three years. He holds the Health Fitness Specialist Certification from the American College of Sports Medicine, is a Certified Strength and Conditioning Specialist through the National Strength and Conditioning Association, and is a National Coach through USA Weightlifting. He has received the College of Health and Human Performance Ray Martinez Teaching Excellence Award.

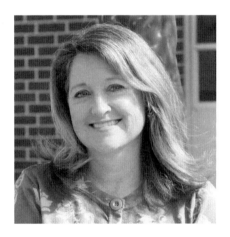

Rhonda Kenny is an instructor in the Department of Kinesiology at East Carolina University, and Director and Internship Coordinator for the Health Fitness Specialist degree program. She holds a BA degree in Physical Education from the University of North Carolina at Chapel Hill and a MAEd in Physical Education from East Carolina University. Mrs. Kenny is a licensed physical education teacher and has experience in fitness club and wellness center management. She teaches Exercise Leadership and holds the Health Fitness Specialist certification from the American College of Sports Medicine, and is a certified group fitness instructor through the Aerobics and Fitness Association of America (AFAA). Mrs. Kenny received the College of Health and Human Performance Ray Martinez Teaching Excellence Award. She was recognized by East Carolina University as one of 10 faculty across campus receiving the highest number of student votes for "The person at ECU who made the most significant positive contribution to a student's education."

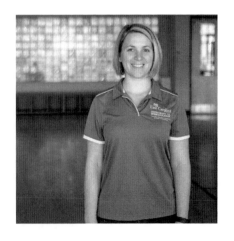

Susan L. Cohen is an instructor in the Department of Kinesiology at East Carolina University and is the director of the Lifetime Physical Activity and Fitness Program. She holds a BS degree in Applied Physiology and Kinesiology from the University of Florida and an MA in Sports and Fitness from the University of Central Florida. Mrs. Cohen holds several group fitness and personal training certifications including Certified Exercise Physiologist from the American College of Sports Medicine. Prior to joining the faculty at East Carolina University, she worked in strength and conditioning, corporate and commercial fitness as well campus recreation at the University of South Florida. Sue-L supervises graduate students who teach within the Department of Kinesiology.

MODULE ONE

WELCOME TO KINE 1000 – YOUR FIRST STEP TO A LIFETIME OF WELLNESS

Dear KINE 1000 Student:

Have you ever been working out or exercising and had the feeling that you didn't belong? Have you ever played a sport and felt you weren't as good as the other players? Do you look around and convince yourself that everyone else is more fit than you? Do you feel uncomfortable walking into the Student Recreation Center? If you answered yes to any of these questions, then you are right where you belong.

You are not competing against anyone else in your class; you are completing against stress... and other health related issues.

A physically active lifestyle is associated with many positive health and performance benefits. As you will learn from this class—Fitness Matters! Our goal is to provide you with the knowledge, skills, and ability to lead an active and healthy lifestyle and help you find activities you enjoy.

We recognize that all of you are in different places in terms of your physical activity habits. Some of you may be fitness fanatics while others may be athletes or former athletes striving to make the change from being involved in competitive sport to an exerciser. Others of you may currently be inactive but want to get into an exercise routine. Finally, some of you may not enjoy being active and are not really sure why you should start an exercise program.

This class is designed to provide you with an in-depth understanding of the importance of being physically active now and in the years to come. Throughout the semester you will develop an understanding of why being physically active is important for both your physical and mental health.

In addition to providing information on the benefits of an active lifestyle, this class will also provide you with the tools to lead an active lifestyle if you choose to do so. You will learn how to design your own exercise program that will help you achieve your health and fitness goals. Throughout the semester you will have the chance to develop motivational skills that will help you stick with your exercise program.

While you will experience many different learning activities throughout the semester, it is important for you to understand the importance of getting accurate fitness baseline information to develop greater self-awareness. A portion of the class will include assessments of your body composition, aerobic fitness, flexibility, strength and endurance.

The information from the assessments will let you know how you compare to health-related standards. For some of you, these assessments will confirm that you are active and fit. For others, some of your information might not be what you expected. You might be heavier than you want to be, your aerobic fitness level might be lower than is needed for health benefits, or you might not be as strong as you thought you were. Regardless of how you score on the assessments, the purpose is to provide you with a starting point for making lifestyle changes.

This is an exploratory class; we want you to learn about your fitness and health and learn what you can do to maintain or improve in these areas. Above all else, we want you to learn that being physically active can be fun and is an important component of living life fully because **Fitness Matters**.

Sincerely,

The Authors

MODULE TWO

WHY DO WE TAKE FITNESS TESTS?

OBJECTIVES

- Identify the purpose of fitness tests.
- Understand how to use fitness tests to evaluate your fitness status.

INTRODUCTION

The purpose of fitness testing is to provide you with a starting point for making lifestyle changes. Physical fitness is a set of attributes that are related to your ability to be physically active. In this course you will undergo a series of health-related physical fitness tests. As you will learn later in this course, healthy physical fitness levels are associated with many physical and mental health benefits, including weight loss and improved brain function.

The main purpose of fitness testing is to improve your health and performance. For personal meaning, fitness tests are used for goal setting, preparing for specific tasks (such as running a 5K fun run, playing an intramural soccer game, or completing a triathlon), and making plans for improvement. Participation in fitness testing increases self-awareness. Many students report that it feels good to get positive feedback on their fitness. Results that don't meet your expectations can motivate you to make positive changes to your lifestyle. Because this course is designed to empower you to make healthy lifestyle changes, it is important to have baseline scores by which to evaluate these changes.

We encourage you to provide your best effort when completing the fitness tests so that you can meaningfully evaluate your fitness status. We will show you how to compare your fitness test scores to health-related standards. This will help you interpret what your fitness test scores mean and provide information about your health status.

The fitness tests you take will help you evaluate your aerobic fitness, body composition, muscular strength, muscular endurance, and flexibility. After you receive your fitness test results, you will compare your results to health-related standards. If your test results for a given fitness test exceed health-related standards, then you are in the Healthy Fitness Zone. Fitness scores in the Healthy Fitness Zone represent a level of performance that provides some degree of protection from diseases, such as heart disease, stroke, and diabetes.

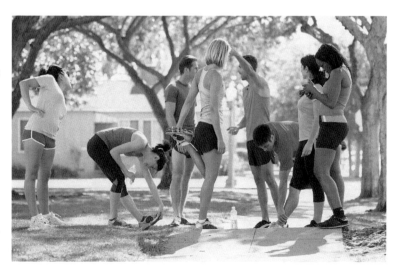

FITNESS MATTERS: SUCCESS STORIES

WHAT STUDENTS SAY ABOUT THIS CLASS . . . .

I was able to increase all skills on the skills test by the end of the semester. — Jenna N.

I enjoyed the skills testing. Honestly, with all these it was just cool to learn a little bit more about exercise and how it can be quantified, its effects, and lifestyle information. — Kyle P.

The skills testing motivated me to continue my workouts because I could see my improvement. — Heather K.

If your fitness test scores fall below the Healthy Fitness Zone, then your test results indicate that some lifestyle changes may improve that area of fitness. Fitness levels far below the health-related standards may indicate an increased health risk.

Your initial fitness test scores will help develop awareness of where you stand relative to health-related standards. This may fuel your motivation to keep doing what you are doing well and create a desire to make healthy lifestyle changes to improve fitness in the areas that are not where you would like them to be. Throughout the semester we will practice skills such as self-monitoring, goal setting, planning, and problem solving to overcome barriers to physical activity. These skills provide the foundation for increasing your

physical activity levels, which can lead to improved fitness and to a better overall sense of well-being.

SUMMARY

Fitness tests increase self-awareness, allow you to set meaningful goals, prepare for particular events, and make specific plans for improvement. The Healthy Fitness Zone represents a level of performance that provides some degree of protection from diseases caused by inactivity and can be used to determine whether you have an adequate level of fitness or whether you need to improve your fitness levels. Your initial fitness test scores provide baseline values so you can determine how much your fitness improves over the course of the semester.

MODULE THREE
PHYSICAL FITNESS TESTING

OBJECTIVES

- Understand how the components of physical fitness are measured.
- Provide opportunities for students to evaluate their own aerobic fitness.

INTRODUCTION

Fitness testing is conducted at the beginning of the semester to allow you the opportunity to set goals and make specific plans for improvement. Your initial fitness test scores provide baseline values so you can determine how much your fitness improves over the course of the semester. Components of health-related physical fitness include aerobic fitness, body composition, muscular strength, muscular endurance, and flexibility. Understanding your current level of fitness, developing your skills for self-assessment, and realizing how good you will feel can inspire you to make changes to improve your fitness levels.

DESCRIPTION OF PHYSICAL FITNESS TESTS

Brief descriptions of physical fitness tests that you will complete in this class are provided below.

ASSESSMENT OF AEROBIC FITNESS

The tests used to assess aerobic fitness in this module are the PACER 20-meter multistage shuttle run and the non-exercise model. An alternative test used to assess aerobic fitness, the mile run, is described in Appendix D.

PACER. The PACER is a multistage 20-meter shuttle run. The objective is to run as long as possible at a specified pace. The participant runs from one side of the course to the other side (20 meters apart) while maintaining the pace set by an audio file. The pace gets faster each minute. Run as long as possible until you can no longer keep pace with the audio file.

PROCEDURES FOR THE PACER

1. Warm-up appropriately. Begin with low-intensity activity, such as walking or slow jogging, designed to increase blood flow to the muscles that you will be using.

2. Have a partner ready to count your laps. The number of laps completed is used to estimate your aerobic fitness.

3. Begin the test when indicated to do so by running across the 20-meter area to the cone on the other side. At the sound of the beep, turn and run back in the other direction across the 20-meter area. If you arrive at the cone before the beep, then wait until the beep before continuing in the other direction.

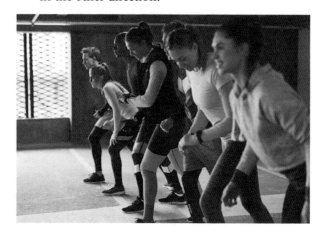

TABLE 3.1

AEROBIC FITNESS TESTING

Name_____ Gender_____ Age _____

Height (feet and inches) _____ Weight (pounds) _____

MEN

Test	Healthy Fitness Zone	Your Score	Healthy Fitness Zone (Yes/No)
PACER (# laps)	≥ 54	_____	_____
Non-Exercise Model VO$_2$ max (mL·kg^{-1}·min^{-1})	≥ 44.3	_____	_____

WOMEN

Test	Healthy Fitness Zone	Your Score	Healthy Fitness Zone (Yes/No)
PACER (# laps)	≥ 38	_____	_____
Non-Exercise Model VO$_2$ max (mL·kg^{-1}·min^{-1})	≥ 38.6	_____	_____

4. Continue to maintain the pace set by the PACER until you can no longer keep up the pace. You are allowed to catch up with the pace until you cannot maintain the pace for two beeps. When you can no longer keep pace with the audio file, the test is ended and you should record the number of laps you completed.

5. Upon completion of the test, cool down for as long as necessary with slow jogging and/or walking (usually for 4 to 7 minutes). Then perform some stretching exercises. Do not sit or lie down immediately after the test. Sitting immediately after heavy exertion can allow the blood to pool in the legs and make you lightheaded.

6. Record the number of laps completed in Table 3.1. Compare your number of laps completed to the standards provided in Table 3.1. Indicate whether your score is greater than or equal to the score required to reach the Healthy Fitness Zone or whether your score indicates the need for improvement.

The PACER is a maximal test, and thus should only be attempted by young and healthy individuals. The test should not be used with individuals who have symptoms of heart disease, such as chest discomfort that results from physical exertion.

The items needed to conduct the test are a flat surface at least 20 meters in length, the PACER audio file, a CD or MP3 player, cones to mark the 20-meter length, and a score sheet on which to record the number of laps performed.

ASSESSMENT OF BODY COMPOSITION

Body Mass Index (BMI). BMI is a weight per height index calculated by dividing weight in kilograms (kg) by the square of height in meters (m). BMI is often used to categorize a person as obese, overweight, normal weight, or underweight. BMI is calculated with the following formula:

$$BMI = weight\ (kg) \div height2\ (m)$$

Procedures to calculate BMI:

1. Divide your weight in pounds by 2.2 to get weight in kilograms.

2. Multiply your height in inches by 0.0254 to get height in meters.

3. Square your height in meters.

4. Divide weight in kilograms (from #1) by the square of height in meters (from #3).

5. Record your BMI in Table 3.2. Compare your BMI to the standards provided in Table 3.2. Indicate whether your BMI is in the Healthy Fitness Zone.

Example: Calculate BMI for a person who weighs 154 pounds and is 5 feet 9 inches tall (i.e., 69 inches).

1. Weight in kilograms = 154 pounds ÷ 2.2 = 70 kg.

2. Height in meters = 69 inches x 0.0254 = 1.7526 m.

3. Squared height in meters = 1.7526 m x 1.7526 m = 3.0716 m^2.

4. BMI = 70 kg ÷ 3.0716 m^2 = 22.79 kg/m^2.

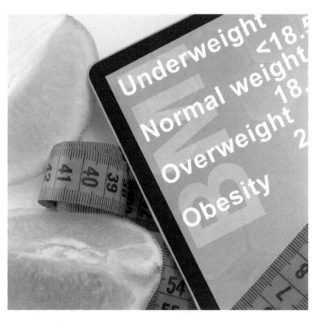

Compute your BMI:

1. Your body weight _____ pounds ÷ 2.2 = kg

2. Your height _____ inches x 0.0254 = m

3. Square your height _____ m x m = m^2

4. Divide line 1 by line 3 = BMI (kg/m^2)

5. Determine if your BMI falls into the Healthy Fitness Zone.

Bioelectrical Impedance Analysis (BIA). Numerous techniques are available to assess body fat levels. One of the newer technologies being used is bioelectrical impedance analysis. BIA is a popular method because it is fast, non-invasive, and, if guidelines are followed, it is an accurate way to determine body fat levels.

BIA depends on hydration status. Results of BIA are more accurate if a person is hydrated than if he or she is dehydrated. If your body fat level is determined via BIA while you are dehydrated, then your body fat level will tend to be overestimated.

To guarantee good results it is important that you adhere to the following guidelines before the assessment:

• Nothing to eat or drink except water for 4 hours prior to the BIA test.

• However, drink plenty of water 4 hours prior to the BIA test.

• No exercise for a minimum of 12 hours prior to the BIA test.

• No alcohol consumption for 48 hours prior to the BIA test.

If you adhere to the guidelines above, then the body fat level recorded from the hand-held Omron testing device should provide a fairly accurate estimate of percent fat. Other factors that can affect your results are certain medications (e.g., diuretics). If you take a diuretic please don't stop taking it. Discuss this with your physician before making changes with any prescription medications. Accuracy of BIA results could also be compromised for women who might be retaining water during the menstrual cycle.

One final note: Make certain you are well hydrated, which means drink plenty of water before the assessment. One way to determine if you're hydrated is to look at the color of your urine. If it is dark yellow, as opposed to light yellow, then you are probably dehydrated, which will result in an overestimation of your body fat level. So drink up, water that is.

ASSESSMENT OF MUSCULAR STRENGTH, ENDURANCE, AND FLEXIBILITY

Curl-up Test. The curl-up test is a measure of abdominal endurance. The objective of this test is to perform as many curl-ups as possible at a specified pace.

PROCEDURES FOR THE CURL-UP TEST

- Lie in a supine position (i.e., on your back on the mat) with your knees bent so that your feet are flat on the floor. Your arms should be straight, by your side, and reaching down toward your feet with the palms facing down.

- Curl-up slowly while sliding your fingers across the mat to the other side of the measuring tape (your fingers must slide forward 4.5 inches on each curl-up). The heels must remain in contact with the mat throughout the curl-up.

- Curl back down until your head touches the mat.

- The curl-up movement is made to a specified cadence of one curl-up every 3 seconds (20 curl-ups per minute). A pre-recorded cadence is used to help you maintain the appropriate pace.

- The score is the number of curl-ups that are performed correctly without pausing.

Push-up Test. The push-up test is a measure of upper body strength and endurance. This is an activity that requires no equipment and can be performed for conditioning and testing purposes throughout your life. The objective of the push-up test is to perform as many push-ups as possible at a specified pace.

PROCEDURES FOR THE PUSH-UP TEST

- Assume a prone (face down) position on the mat. Your hands should be placed under your shoulders, with fingers spread, and legs straight and slightly apart.

TABLE 3.2

BODY COMPOSITION TESTS

Name_____ Gender_____ Age _____

Height (feet and inches) _____ Weight (pounds) _____

MEN

Test	Healthy Fitness Zone	Your Score
Percent Fat (%) [BIA]	7.0 – 22.2	_____
Body Mass Index (kg/m²)	18.3 – 25.1	_____

WOMEN

Test	Healthy Fitness Zone	Your Score
Percent Fat (%) [BIA]	16.5 – 31.3	_____
Body Mass Index (kg/m²)	17.6 – 25.1	_____

- Push up off the mat until your arms are straight. The legs and back should remain straight throughout the entire push-up.

- Then lower your body until the elbows are bent at a 90-degree angle. At this point, the upper arms will usually be parallel to the floor.

- The pushup movement is made to a specified cadence of one push-up every 3 seconds (20 push-ups per minute). A pre-recorded cadence is used to help you maintain the appropriate pace.

- The score is the number of push-ups that are performed correctly without pausing.

- Record the number of curl-ups completed in Table 3.3. Compare the number of curl-ups you completed to the standards provided in Table 3.3. Indicate whether your score is greater than or equal to the score required to reach the Healthy Fitness Zone or whether your score indicates the need for improvement.

PROCEDURES FOR THE SIT-AND-REACH TEST

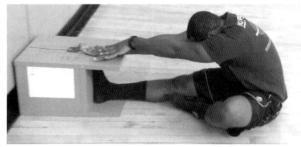

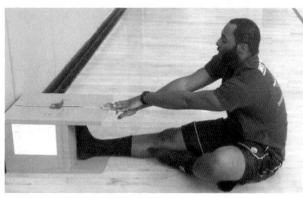

East Carolina University Department of Kinesiology

- Remove your shoes and sit with one foot flat against the sit-and-reach box and that leg fully extended. The other knee should be bent and that foot placed flat on the floor near the side of the knee that is extended. The bent knee can be moved to the side of the body during the movement as needed.

- Place one hand on top of the other and slowly extend the arms forward over the measuring scale. The hands should reach forward evenly.

- Reach slowly forward four times and on the fourth reach hold the position for one second. The knee of the extended leg should remain straight throughout the test.

- After measuring one side, switch the positions of the legs and measure the other side in the same fashion.

- Record the number of push-ups completed in Table 3.3. Compare the number of push-ups you completed to the standards provided in Table 3.3. Indicate whether your score is greater than or equal to the score required to reach the Healthy Fitness Zone or whether your score indicates the need for improvement.

PROCEDURES FOR THE SHOULDER STRETCH TEST

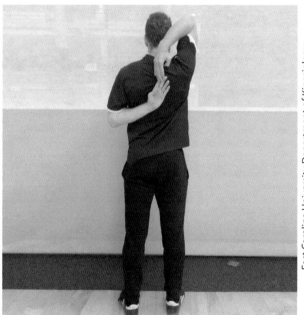

East Carolina University Department of Kinesiology

- Test each side separately. For the right shoulder, reach the right hand over the right shoulder and the left hand behind the back reaching up. For the left shoulder, reach the left hand over the left shoulder and the right hand behind the back reaching up.

- Try to touch the fingers of the right and left hand.

- If you are able to touch the fingers together behind the back, then record a "Yes" in the appropriate place in Table 3.3. If you are unable to touch the fingers together behind the back, then record a "No" in the appropriate place in Table 3.3.

- Inability to touch the fingers together behind the back may indicate the need for improvement of flexibility in the shoulder joint.

SUMMARY

The PACER is a maximal test of aerobic fitness. This means that maximal exertion is needed to perform this test correctly. Percent fat can be estimated from bioelectrical impedance analysis. Muscular strength and endurance can be evaluated with curl-up and push-up tests. These exercises are also appropriate activities to help you maintain fitness throughout your life. Flexibility can be assessed with the sit-and-reach and shoulder stretch tests. Your initial fitness tests will provide you with baseline values so you can determine how much your fitness improves over the course of the semester. Now that you have this crucial information about your fitness levels, we will focus on why fitness matters and what's in it for you.

FITNESS MATTERS: SUCCESS STORIES

WHAT STUDENTS SAY ABOUT THIS CLASS . . . .

When I did the skills testing at the beginning of the semester, I realized that I was so out of shape. Throughout the semester, I decided to start working out for 30 minutes a few times a week and this class helped me do that. I am making my own workout plan and I also do yoga. I do these at least 3 or 4 times a week. — Heather H.

Skills testing allowed me to identify that while my muscular strength is adequate, my ability to perform aerobic exercise needs work. — Alex B.

I have been able to assess my strengths and weaknesses with skills testing. Pushing myself beyond my thought-to-be limits has helped me with my self-confidence and dedication to an exercise program. — Bobby Jo J.

TABLE 3.3

MUSCULAR STRENGTH, MUSCULAR ENDURANCE, AND FLEXIBILITY TESTS

MEN

Test	Healthy Fitness Zone	Your Score	Healthy Fitness Zone (Yes/No)
Abdominal Strength and Endurance			
Curl-ups (# completed) ≥ 24	_____	_____	_____
Upper Body Strength and Endurance			
Push-ups (# completed) ≥ 18	_____	_____	_____
Flexibility			
Sit-and-Reach (inches)			
Right leg 8	_____	_____	_____
Left leg 8	_____	_____	_____
Shoulder Stretch			
Right Side Touch fingers together behind back	_____	_____	_____
Left Side	_____	_____	_____

WOMEN

Test	Healthy Fitness Zone	Your Score	Healthy Fitness Zone (Yes/No)
Abdominal Strength and Endurance			
Curl-ups (# completed) ≥ 18	_____	_____	_____
Upper Body Strength and Endurance			
Push-ups (# completed) ≥ 7	_____	_____	_____
Modified Pull-ups (# completed) ≥ 4	_____	_____	_____
Flexibility			
Sit-and-Reach (inches)			
Right leg 12	_____	_____	_____
Left leg 12	_____	_____	_____
Shoulder Stretch			
Right Side Touch fingers together behind back	_____	_____	_____
Left Side	_____	_____	_____

MODULE FOUR

REASONS FOR EXERCISE: WHAT'S IN IT FOR YOU?

OBJECTIVES

- Understand the benefits of leading an active lifestyle.
- Develop greater self-awareness of your personal reasons for being active and how being active may potentially benefit you.

INTRODUCTION

If exercise could be packed into a pill, it would be the most beneficial and widely prescribed medication on the market. It is pretty remarkable that every single system (e.g., skeletal, muscular, cardiovascular, respiratory, metabolic, immune, brain) in our body benefits from an active lifestyle.

Not only is physical activity participation associated with increased physical health and well-being, it is also associated with numerous mental health benefits. Physical activity plays an important role in stress management, and is associated with decreased anxiety and depression along with improved quality of life. An active lifestyle can improve self-esteem. Students report that being active helps them feel good about themselves and provides a sense of accomplishment. Physical activity can also improve mood and concentration. Both vigorous physical activities designed to develop cardiovascular fitness and moderate intensity lifestyle activities have important physical and mental health benefits.

Many people are aware that participating in physical activity is good for them, yet fail to lead an active lifestyle. Approximately 60% of the population does not achieve the recommended amount of physical activity and approximately 40% of the population is sedentary. Of those who start a program, many unfortunately, don't succeed at staying active. Typically, 50% of all individuals who start an exercise program discontinue within six months. Most of the dropouts occur within the first month or two. If students can get through the first few months, they are more likely to stay active. Or if they do temporarily stop being active, they are likely to restart a program because being active becomes a habit and part of their lifestyle and identity.

Like the general population, there is great variability in student activity levels. You might already enjoy being active and view an active lifestyle as part of who you are and your self-identity. Others might recognize the importance of being active, but have difficulty finding the motivation to exercise. Some of you might not have bought into the importance of leading an active lifestyle. The purpose of this module is to help you explore the reasons why you might want to be active.

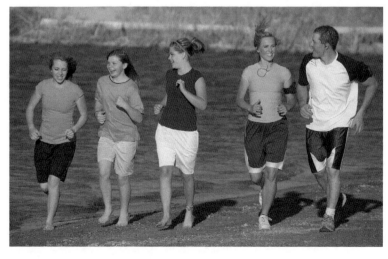

WEIGHING THE PROS AND CONS OF BEING ACTIVE

The first step on the journey to an active lifestyle is to consider the pros and cons of being active. Do you know what benefits you'd like to receive from an active lifestyle? Have you thought about what your lifestyle would be like if you were physically active? Have you made increasing your physical activity a priority? If you answered yes to these questions, you may already lead an active lifestyle or perhaps be ready to make the commitment to being active. If you answered no or are unsure at this point, you might benefit from completing a decision balance sheet. Completing the decision balance sheet that follows should help you weigh the pros and cons of leading an active lifestyle.

What did you notice after completing the decision balance sheet? You may have discovered more pros than cons to being active. Alternatively, you may have noticed some pros to being active, but also some cons or barriers to being active. If you noted mostly long-term benefits such as improved health or weight loss, are there any short-term reasons for being active (e.g., improved mood, increased energy, better sleep quality, decreased stress or simply to have fun)? Are there benefits that connect to your life values and things that are important to you? If you are currently inactive or struggling with motivation, leading an active lifestyle can certainly be challenging. Although the process of adjusting to a new way of living can be eased into, it is hardly ever easy. Throughout this semester we hope to provide you with skills and abilities that you can use to overcome the negatives associated with an active lifestyle. We also encourage you to revisit your decision balance sheet throughout the semester as you may become aware of some additional personally important benefits that you may not have initially realized. Some of the cons you

DECISION BALANCE SHEET

Instructions: List the pros and cons to becoming more physically active in the appropriate boxes.

Gains to Self (Pros)	Losses to Self (Cons)
• More energy	• Less time to do other "fun" things
• Weight loss	• Don't like the feelings associated with exercise
•	•
•	•
•	•
Gains to Important Others	**Losses to Important Others**
• More attractive to significant others	• Less time with friends
• Can play sports with my friends	•
•	•
•	•
•	•
Self-Approval	**Self-Disapproval**
• Feel more confident	• Feel intimidated at recreation center
• Feel better about myself knowing I'm doing something good for myself	• Feel awkward because I'm out of shape
•	•
•	•

noted today may become less important while you may also become aware of some additional roadblocks to an active lifestyle. Another strategy that may help develop greater self-awareness and insights on what kind of activities you may enjoy is to reflect on the reasons for being active.

REASONS TO BE PHYSICALLY ACTIVE

Exercise motives are the reasons people give for exercise. If you ask college students why they started a physical activity program, they will most often mention health/fitness and appearance reasons. They might state that, "I started my program to lose weight, to look better, and to improve my health." No doubt, improving and maintaining health and fitness are important motivators. However, are those reasons strong enough motivators to keep a person active? For many people the answer is "no."

Students who exercise simply to improve how they look and to get fit often do not succeed at sticking with an active lifestyle. Those reasons for being active are associated with low success because they are very outcome-oriented reasons and associated with future benefits. As much as our culture likes quick results and as much as we would like to see instant changes in health, fitness, and weight, those changes do not occur overnight. What is the solution? Find activities that you enjoy. If we compare students who are active and inactive, we see that both groups are similar in that they initiate a physical activity program to improve their health, fitness, and appearance. However, those who stay active still value the health and fitness benefits, but they also place importance on enjoyment-related reasons for being active. In a nutshell, those who continue exercise programs report that they enjoy physical activity more than those who do not. It is rare for people to continue to be active unless they find the experience enjoyable and meaningful.

Exercising solely for health/fitness reasons can lack personal meaning and purpose. Walking/running on a treadmill or riding an exercise bike to nowhere seems pointless to some. These activity modes depict images of a "workout" that seem like all work and no fun. However, these individuals may find commuting via bicycle or foot, playing sports, training for a race, or walking a dog to have personal significance and intrinsic meaning.

A key strategy in developing an active lifestyle is to choose activities you enjoy. Some students really enjoy the social aspects of physical activity and the chance to hang out with friends. If social interaction makes physical activity fun for you, workout with a friend. Other people like the chance for some "me time," and the opportunity to reflect on things going on in their lives while exercising. If that sounds like you, choose activities that offer time for solitude.

> ### K E Y   P O I N T
> In addition to developing fitness, do not overlook the importance of choosing activities that allow you to obtain other enjoyable outcomes.

Other people participate in physical activity because they enjoy doing an activity they are good at, or they enjoy the challenge of learning and improving their skills. While others yet enjoy the process of competing or the sensations they have while doing the activity, such as the feeling they have when they make a great shot in tennis or the feelings they have while swimming. If that sounds like you, pick an activity that gives you those positive feelings. Participate in club or intramural sports if competition stimulates you. Some of you might be adrenaline junkies. If that is the case, pick activities that provide a sense of excitement. Others yet may find physical activity more gratifying if they are training for a purpose – if that is the case, training for a road race or triathlon may be the ticket. An important, but often overlooked, ingredient to an active lifestyle is to find activities that you personally enjoy.

Although choosing an enjoyable activity probably seems intuitive, many students fail to do so. If you are not sure which activities you would like best, sample a variety of activities. Through sampling, you will discover which activities are the most fun and help improve your mood. Learn new skills when your routine starts to get boring. If you find riding an exercise bike boring, or if you dislike swimming, or feel awkward at aerobics, but love to play basketball and soccer – choose basketball and soccer!

To help clarify why you want to exercise, take a moment to fill out the participation motivation questionnaire titled, "Physical Activity: What's In It For Me?" Following this questionnaire, you'll write a list of activities that are compatible with your motivation. In selecting activities, make sure to choose activities that are compatible with what you want to receive from physical activity participation.

One note: There are no right or wrong answers in this questionnaire. Rather, the questionnaire is for your information only. So be honest! What's in it for you?

SUMMARY

Physical activity participation is an important component of stress management and is associated with decreased anxiety and depression. Students also report that physical activity makes them feel better and improves their mood. In this module, you received information to help you recognize the benefits of leading an active lifestyle and develop greater self-awareness of your personal reasons for being active.

Believing in the importance of physical activity and finding activities that you enjoy are the first steps on the journey to an active lifestyle.

PHYSICAL ACTIVITY: WHAT'S IN IT FOR ME?

Rate how important each of the following incentives or reasons for participating in physical activity is for you personally. Why do you want to lead an active lifestyle?

	Not at all important			Very Important	
To improve my health	1	2	3	④	5
To improve my physical fitness	1	2	3	④	5
To lose or manage my weight	1	2	3	4	⑤
To improve my muscle tone/strength	1	2	③	4	5
To look better	1	2	3	4	⑤
To feel better	1	2	3	4	⑤
To reduce stress	1	2	③	4	5
Because I enjoy being active	1	②	3	4	5
To have fun	1	②	3	4	5
Because I enjoy the social camaraderie	1	②	3	4	5
Because I enjoy competition	1	②	3	4	5
To experience thrills and excitement	1	②	3	4	5
To challenge myself	1	2	③	4	5
Because I enjoy improving and mastering fitness/sport skills	1	②	3	4	5
To have the chance to put things in perspective	1	②	3	4	5
Because I like the sensations I experience while doing the activity	1	②	3	4	5
Because I enjoy getting absorbed in the activity	1	②	3	4	5
Because I enjoy doing things at which I'm successful	1	②	3	4	5

If you circled a "4" or a "5" for an item, then you consider that item an important reason to be physically active. Now list different activities that are compatible with the reasons why you personally want to exercise.

-Zumba
-stationary bike
-treadmil
-weight lifting

FITNESS MATTERS: SUCCESS STORIES

WHAT STUDENTS SAY ABOUT THIS CLASS . . . .

I learned how to start an exercise program that I can stick to and how to focus on activities I enjoy. I enjoy yoga and ZUMBA™. — Kinzey P.

I learned a lot about my own body and what I specifically need to do to improve and accomplish my goals. I love using the bikes upstairs while doing homework. It's a good way to do physical activity and be productive at the same time. — Anna H.

They have really shown me all the different options I have for exercise. It doesn't have to be boring! I participate in core training—I love doing that! — Tatum G.

MODULE FIVE

PHYSICAL ACTIVITY, FITNESS, AND HEALTH BENEFITS FOR COLLEGE STUDENTS

OBJECTIVES

- Identify the health benefits of regular physical activity.
- Understand that regular physical activity can impact mental health, as well as physical health.

INTRODUCTION

Regular physical activity will help you feel better and improve your health. Because of the ability of the human brain to take a behavior and turn it into an automatic routine, the habits you develop as a college student can carry over to the rest of your life. The information you learn from this book will help you understand the importance of physical activity for health. We provide you with information regarding the benefits of physical activity and exercise on physical health and mental health, specific suggestions for improving physical fitness, and ways to develop the skills and abilities needed to adopt and maintain a healthy lifestyle. We hope you decide to use this information to be active, fit, and healthy for the rest of your life.

This module is about physical activity, exercise, fitness, and health. What do these terms mean, how do they differ, and why are they important? First, let's define a few terms.

Physical Activity. Physical activity is any body movement produced by skeletal muscles that result in a substantial increase in energy expenditure.

Energy Expenditure. Energy expenditure is the number of calories used during normal bodily functions and physical activity.

Exercise. Exercise is physical activity that is planned and structured and requires repetitive movement that is done to improve or maintain one or more aspects of physical fitness.

Physical Fitness. Physical fitness is a set of attributes that relate to the ability to perform physical activity. The components of physical fitness related to health include aerobic fitness, body composition, muscular strength, muscular endurance, and flexibility. Each of these components will be examined in other modules.

From these definitions you should understand that exercise is a type of physical activity and that physical activity includes more than just exercise. For example, walking to class, gardening, taking the stairs instead of the elevator, playing softball, and moving furniture are all forms of physical activity, but might not necessarily

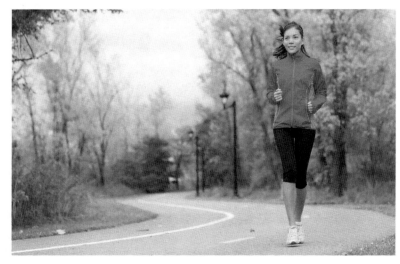

be considered exercise. Regular exercise and adequate levels of physical activity will make you feel better and contribute to improved health.

Just how is physical activity good for you? Let us count the ways:

Regular physical activity:

- Helps some people lose weight
- Helps other people maintain a healthy body weight
- Reduces the risk of heart disease and stroke
- Decreases high blood pressure and the risk of developing high blood pressure
- Increases feelings of psychological well-being
- Reduces feelings of stress
- Builds healthy muscles, bones, and joints
- Decreases the risk of developing type 2 diabetes
- Reduces the risk of colon cancer
- Increases the good cholesterol (high-density lipoproteins [HDL])
- Decreases blood fats (triglycerides)
- Decreases depression and anxiety

A few more reasons to be physically active:

- The current generation of children in the United States is the first that will have a lower life expectancy than their parents.
- A child born in the year 2000 has a 1 in 3 chance of developing diabetes.
- People who develop obesity or diabetes have a lowered life expectancy of 15 to 20 years.

PHYSICAL ACTIVITY, FITNESS, AND HEALTH

Dr. Ralph Paffenbarger, Jr. was a noted researcher who provided important evidence on the health benefits of physical activity. In two important studies, the San Francisco longshoremen study and the Harvard alumni study, Paffenbarger and his colleagues demonstrated that physical activity is related to heart disease. In both studies, individuals with high levels of energy expenditure (caloric expenditure) had fewer heart attacks. In the Harvard alumni study, the physical activity and heart attack rates of nearly 17,000 men were measured. Men who expended fewer than 500 calories per week through physical activity had the highest heart attack rate. These men would be considered very sedentary. A steady decline in heart attack risk was evidenced as physical activity increased (i.e., more calories were expended) up to a level of 2,000 calories per week. The value of 2,000 calories per week apparently provided close to maximal protection because heart attack risk leveled off at this value.

FITNESS MATTERS: SUCCESS STORIES

WHAT STUDENTS SAY ABOUT THIS CLASS . . . .

This class gave me better insight on a healthy living style not just physically but emotionally, and made me want to maintain a healthy lifestyle and adjust some areas I was lacking in. — Rayleen J.

I think the majority of the concepts we went over this semester have helped me to become more informed about my body and have helped to outline ways I can personally live a healthier lifestyle. I have signed up for two yoga classes over the summer. I also really enjoyed circuit training. It's fast-paced and it allows you to use your own surroundings/everyday items. — Hannah F.

I recently experienced a spinal injury that made it nearly impossible to exercise in any way without pain. My instructor encouraged me to do what I could and at least try, so I did. My injury doesn't bother me as much anymore and now I feel confident that I can live a healthy and happy life. — Elizabeth H.

In another study, Paffenbarger and his colleagues provided an important message for current and former athletes. Having been an athlete does not provide protection from heart disease unless the individual remains physically active. Former athletes and non-athletes who were currently active (i.e., expend ≥ 2,000 calories per week) had the lowest heart attack risk. Former athletes who became sedentary (< 500 calories per week) had the highest heart attack risk (even higher than sedentary non-athletes). The cumulative message from the work of these researchers and of many others is that you can be healthier (lower your risk of cardiovascular disease) if you are physically active enough to expend a sufficient number of calories. Figure 5.1 is a graph of data published by Paffenbarger and his colleagues. This graph clearly shows the inverse relationship between physical activity and death from cardiovascular diseases, coronary heart disease, stroke, and respiratory diseases. This means that as the caloric expenditure from physical activity increased, the death rates from these diseases decreased.

The previous discussion emphasized that regular physical activity can improve health and lower cardiovascular disease risk. What about the effect of aerobic fitness on improved health status and disease risk reduction? It is widely known that increases in physical activity will increase aerobic fitness, but is it the increased aerobic fitness or the physical activity that improves health? Research evidence demonstrates that both physical activity and aerobic fitness are significantly related to mortality.

Dr. Steven Blair demonstrated the importance of aerobic fitness on all-cause mortality (death from all causes, particularly heart disease and cancer). Blair and his colleagues divided a large sample of men and women into five groups based upon aerobic fitness (adjusted for age). They observed that aerobic fitness was related to mortality [see Figure 5.2]. However, the most striking finding was that low aerobic fitness was associated with dramatic increases in mortality. Men and women in the lowest fitness groups were more than three times more likely to die than the people in the other groups. The risk for the highest fitness group was not much lower than the risk for the moderate fitness group, but moving out of the lowest fitness group to the next lowest fitness group was associated with a significant reduction in risk. The value of aerobic fitness needed to reduce mortality risk (i.e., move out of the lowest fitness group) is within reach

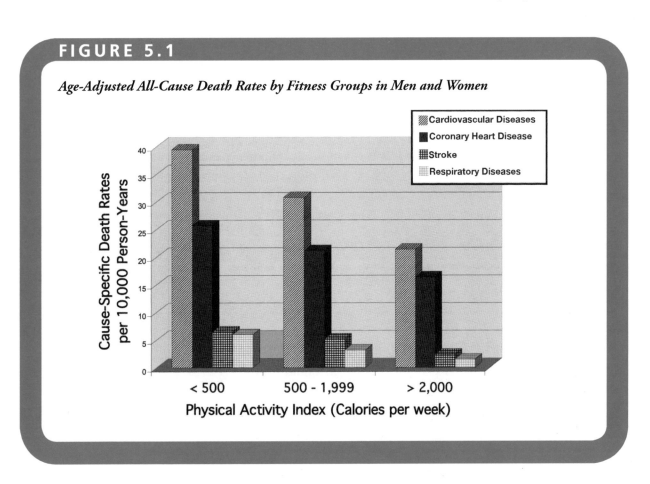

FIGURE 5.1

Age-Adjusted All-Cause Death Rates by Fitness Groups in Men and Women

Legend:
- Cardiovascular Diseases
- Coronary Heart Disease
- Stroke
- Respiratory Diseases

Y-axis: Cause-Specific Death Rates per 10,000 Person-Years

X-axis: Physical Activity Index (Calories per week): < 500, 500 - 1,999, > 2,000

FIGURE 5.2

Cause-Specific Death Rates by Physical Activity Index

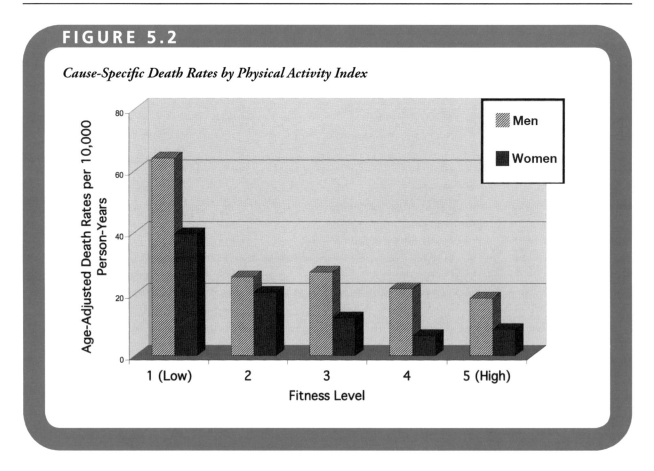

of most individuals who are moderately physically active. For most people, the physical activity needed to reach this level of fitness can be accomplished with a brisk walk each day of 30 to 60 minutes.

In summary, both aerobic fitness and regular physical activity are important for health. If you exercise with sufficient regularity to guarantee moderate levels of physical fitness, you will be healthier and live longer.

PHYSICAL ACTIVITY AND MENTAL HEALTH

A physically active lifestyle is as important for mental health as it is for physical health. In this section, we will discuss the importance of mental health and then highlight the relationship between exercise and mental health.

It is estimated that 20-25% of the population suffers some sort of mental health disorder in any given year. In fact, the majority of hospital beds in the United States are occupied by individuals with mental health issues. Two of the more common mental health disorders are anxiety and depression. These disorders are long-lasting and interfere with normal everyday life functioning. Some estimates suggest that at least

one-third of the population will suffer from at least one bout of depression in their life. The statistics are similar for anxiety disorders. Unfortunately, many individuals who experience mental health disorders do not seek treatment. In fact, only about one-third of the people with depression seek treatment. These percentages emphasize how common mental health problems are in today's society.

Mental health problems are linked to a decreased quality of life and to a variety of physical health problems that include sleeping, eating, sexual, school, alcohol/drug, and interpersonal problems. Increasingly, it is being recognized that many physical diseases are influenced by psychological factors. Mental health problems can influence the onset, progression, and severity of many physical health issues. That the mind affects the body is not a new idea; it at least goes back to Plato, who emphasized the idea of "a sound mind in a sound body." One strategy for improving mental health is to focus on improving one's physical health.

So what can be done to improve mental health? A variety of approaches can be used, such as counseling, stress management, and medication. In addition to these techniques, exercise is increasingly being recognized as an effective tool for improving mental health. Regular exercise may be as effective in helping individuals manage stress and anxiety as traditional stress management techniques. Increasing evidence also shows that exercise may be effective in treating depression. Researchers from Duke University studied 156 patients with a major depressive disorder and compared how effective exercise was to anti-depressant medications.

KEY POINT
Moderate levels of aerobic fitness offer important health benefits. The key is moving from the unfit category to the moderately fit category. Anyone can make this move by walking briskly each day for 30 minutes or more.

Overall, anti-depressant medications were associated with faster symptom relief, but by the end of four months, exercise was as effective as anti-depressant medications in combating depression. Six months after the end of the study, the exercise group had a lower relapse rate compared to those taking anti-depressant medications. Another benefit of using exercise as a treatment is that it is not associated with the negative side effects that accompany medications to treat depression, and the side effects of exercise include improved exercise-related health outcomes.

Although individuals who have the poorest mental health gain the most from exercise, even those with normal mental health levels can benefit. Mental health also includes the presence of positive self-esteem and well-being. Physically active people feel better about themselves compared to less-active people.

Cognitive function is a person's ability in processes like working memory, learning, and comprehension. Numerous research studies have demonstrated that regular exercise leads to enhanced improved cognitive functioning.

There is more good news. Although exercise on a regular basis is important, even a single bout of exercise has short-term mental health benefits. A single session of exercise can lower stress, muscle tension, anxiety, depression, and other negative mood states. It can also increase positive moods and help a person feel invigorated and energized. In fact, college students report that one of the common reasons they exercise is because they feel better and less stressed after a good workout.

SUMMARY

Regular physical activity results in a host of health benefits. Both physical activity and physical fitness are related to death rates and cardiovascular disease risk factors. Physical activity also has positive benefits for mental health.

- People who expend more calories through regular physical activity have lower mortality rates.

- People who are in the lowest aerobic fitness category have substantially higher mortality rates. Moving from the least fit category to a moderately fit category is associated with a dramatic reduction in mortality rates.

- Physical activity is an important component in the treatment of depression, anxiety, and other mood disturbances.

MODULE SIX

AEROBIC FITNESS

OBJECTIVES

- Introduce the concept of aerobic fitness and the factors that influence it.
- Understand the difference between aerobic and anaerobic exercise.
- Understand the units in which aerobic fitness is expressed.
- Understand how aerobic fitness can be measured and estimated.
- Provide opportunities for students to evaluate their own aerobic fitness.

INTRODUCTION

Aerobic fitness is the ability of the heart, lungs, and blood vessels to supply oxygen to the working muscles and the ability of the muscles to utilize oxygen to continue work or exercise. We typically think of aerobic fitness as the ability to perform exercises that use large muscle groups for an extended period. The term "aerobic fitness" is used interchangeably with several other terms, including cardiovascular endurance, cardiorespiratory endurance, aerobic capacity, and maximal oxygen consumption.

Module 5 provided evidence demonstrating that regular physical activity leads to better health (e.g., decreased risk of cardiovascular disease) and that a higher level of aerobic fitness is associated with better health. Physical activity of sufficient intensity that contributes to improved aerobic fitness is generally considered aerobic exercise.

THE AEROBIC VS. ANAEROBIC EXERCISE CONTINUUM

Aerobic means "in the presence of oxygen." Aerobic exercise is exercise that takes place in the presence of sufficient oxygen. Exercises of at least a moderate intensity, such as walking, jogging, and cycling are considered aerobic. This is because sufficient oxygen is available to meet the demands of these exercises. Although the same can be said for activities such as softball, bowling, and golf, these activities are of too

low an intensity and too intermittent to provide the same health benefits. Therefore, the term "aerobic exercise" will refer to exercises that are aerobic in nature that can also produce an increase in aerobic fitness.

Examples of aerobic exercises include walking, jogging/running, elliptical training, swimming, rowing, group fitness classes, cycling, and

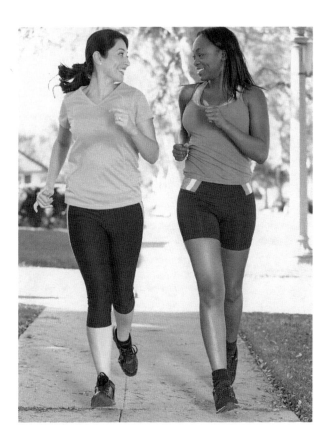

continuous calisthenics. Several popular aerobic exercises can be performed in their natural environment or on machines designed to reproduce the exercise in a more feasible or in a more interesting fashion. These exercises include running on a treadmill, cycling, rowing, cross-country skiing, and stair stepping. Other aerobic exercises, such as group fitness classes, are offered in many Student Recreation Centers or can be done at home with a DVD. Several sports (e.g., basketball, racquetball, tennis) can provide gains in aerobic fitness and can be considered aerobic exercises if they are performed at an appropriate intensity for sufficient periods.

Anaerobic means "in the absence of oxygen." Exercises that are considered anaerobic are usually of a high intensity so that sufficient oxygen is not available to meet the oxygen demand. When the oxygen supply is insufficient, waste products, such as lactic acid, accumulate and limit the duration of the exercise. Activities that have a high anaerobic component include sprinting, weight lifting, calisthenics, and many sports. Several activities can be classified as aerobic if performed continuously at lower intensities or as anaerobic if performed for short periods at higher intensities (e.g., basketball, swimming, running). Most activities require use of both aerobic and anaerobic metabolism. As such, exercises should be thought of along an aerobic-anaerobic continuum.

The traditional way to improve aerobic fitness has involved continuous activity at low to moderate intensities. However, recent research has indicated that short bouts of higher intensity training with periods of rest separating the short bouts (i.e., interval training) can increase aerobic fitness as well. One possible benefit of performing interval training over the continuous training methods is that the duration needed for interval training is significantly less.

KEY POINT
Aerobic exercises use large muscle groups and can be done continuously. Participation in regular aerobic exercise will produce increases in aerobic fitness.

THE BEST INDEX OF AEROBIC FITNESS: VO_2 MAX

Maximal oxygen consumption (VO_2 max) is widely recognized as the most valid index of aerobic fitness. VO_2 max is the maximal amount of oxygen one is able to use during maximal exercise. VO_2 max can be expressed in several units. In absolute terms, VO_2 max can be expressed as liters of oxygen per minute ($L\cdot min^{-1}$) or milliliters of oxygen per minute ($mL\cdot min^{-1}$). When it is important to take into account one's body weight (i.e., whenever the body weight is moved, such as when running), VO_2 max is typically expressed as milliliters of oxygen per kilogram of body weight per minute ($mL\cdot kg^{-1}\cdot min^{-1}$). It is useful to become familiar with VO_2 max values expressed in this fashion so that you can interpret your own level of aerobic fitness. World-class male endurance runners, who are highly fit, have VO_2 max values in the 70s and higher. World-class female endurance runners have VO_2 max values in the 60s and higher. The average college-age male will probably have a VO_2 max between 41 and 46 $mL\cdot kg^{-1}\cdot min^{-1}$. The average college-age female will have a VO_2 max close to 40 $mL\cdot kg^{-1}\cdot min^{-1}$.

KEY POINT
VO_2 max is the best index of aerobic fitness and is expressed in relative terms as milliliters of oxygen per kilogram of body weight per minute ($mL\cdot kg^{-1}\cdot min^{-1}$). By expressing VO_2 max in these terms, it is easy to determine one's relative aerobic fitness level, and comparisons can be made between people who differ on body weight.

INFLUENCE OF AGE, HEREDITY, GENDER, AND PHYSICAL ACTIVITY LEVEL ON VO_2 MAX

It is well documented that we become less fit as we age. After age 30 the typical decline in VO_2 max is about 0.3 $mL\cdot kg^{-1}\cdot min^{-1}$ per year. This represents a decline of about 1% per year. If you begin or continue to train aerobically, the decline in VO_2 max with age is lessened. Research indicates that habitual physical activity has a greater effect on aerobic capacity than does chronological age.

Studies on identical and fraternal twins indicate a substantial genetic effect on VO_2 max. This may mean that unless you have the "right" genes you will never become a world-class distance runner, but it does not mean that you cannot improve your personal fitness level. Although the response to training is hard to predict because it is in large part genetically determined, it is estimated that previously sedentary individuals can improve their VO_2 max by about 20%, although larger increases in VO_2 max have been reported. Your initial fitness level must be kept in mind when evaluating improvements in VO_2 max. A greater degree of improvement can be expected from previously sedentary individuals than from individuals who are more highly trained and thus closer to their genetic potential.

Initial fitness level and genetic differences influence the amount of improvement in fitness one will experience with exercise training. Lower fit individuals can show a greater percentage improvement when compared to higher fit individuals. However, individual responses differ greatly. As much as 50% of one's ability to improve his or her fitness level is determined by genetics. Thus, some individuals will see substantial improvements with training, whereas other with similar fitness levels will show smaller changes. Because of these differences, individuals are sometimes described as being low, medium, or high exercise responders. Regardless of how one responds, however, it is important to remember that exercise, even without fitness improvements, enhances health. While you might not be able to win a marathon, being physically active can improve your health.

Values of VO_2 max for women are generally 10 to 20% lower than corresponding values for men at a similar age. This gender difference in VO_2 max is probably due to differences in body fat, lean body mass, heart size, and hemoglobin concentration between males and females. The average percent body fat for women is about 37%, while the average for men is about 24%. Since men generally have less body fat, a greater amount of muscle mass, and a larger heart size than women they tend to have a higher aerobic capacity. In addition, men have a greater hemoglobin concentration than women (about 15 mg/dL for men and 13 mg/dL for women). The greater the amount of hemoglobin in the blood, the greater the amount of oxygen the blood can carry.

This means that the oxygen carrying capacity of the blood is greater in men than in women.

Age, heredity, and gender are unalterable factors that affect aerobic capacity. However, physical activity is directly under your control and adherence to a regular exercise program can increase VO_2 max. However, it appears that no two individuals will respond the same way to a given training program. It is difficult to predict precisely how one will respond to increases in aerobic training because the degree of improvement depends upon several factors, including heredity; current state of training; and the intensity, frequency, and duration of the training program.

> ### KEY POINT
> Because of genetic differences, no two people will have the same response to a training program. However, most people can improve their aerobic fitness with the proper intensity, frequency, and duration of training.

MEASUREMENT OF AEROBIC FITNESS

VO_2 max, also called maximal oxygen consumption, is measured through expired gas analysis. Measurement of expired gases is called indirect calorimetry. Measurement of VO_2 max through indirect calorimetry is relatively expensive and requires trained personnel. The individual is required to exercise to exhaustion (usually on a treadmill or cycle ergometer). During this exercise, oxygen consumption, carbon dioxide production, and volume of air are measured with special equipment. Fortunately, actual measurement of VO_2 max through indirect calorimetry is not necessary except in certain circumstances (e.g., research studies). Because oxygen consumption is related to exercise intensity and heart rate response, VO_2 max can be estimated relatively accurately.

ESTIMATION OF VO_2 MAX

Because measurement of VO_2 max is time consuming and expensive, it is often desirable to be able to estimate aerobic fitness. Aerobic fitness can be estimated from one of several methods:

- PACER
- Mile Run
- Non-Exercise Model (from measures taken without exercise testing)

PACER. The PACER is a multistage 20-meter shuttle run. The objective is to run as long as possible at a specified pace. The participant runs from one side of the course to the other side (20 meters apart) while maintaining the pace set by an audio file. The pace gets faster each minute so that eventually less fit participants cannot maintain the pace and must stop running. The more fit participants will be able to maintain the pace for a longer time than the less fit participants.

Results from the PACER can then be compared to the standards in Table 6.1 to determine whether you are in the Healthy Fitness Zone or whether you need improvement in this area. The Healthy Fitness Zone (previously defined in Module 2) represents a level of performance that provides some degree of protection from hypokinetic diseases, such as heart disease, stroke, and diabetes.

Mile Run. The objective of the Mile Run is to cover a 1-mile course as quickly as possible. It is best to pace yourself to maintain a steady relatively fast pace throughout the test. If you are unable to run the entire mile, it is okay to walk, as long as you are covering the distance as quickly as you can.

Based on the time to complete the mile, age, gender, and body mass index (BMI), VO2 max can be estimated. BMI is calculated from weight and height. Results can then be compared to the standards for VO2 max in Table 6.1 to determine whether your aerobic fitness is in the Healthy Fitness Zone.

Non-Exercise Model. Aerobic fitness can be accurately estimated from measures taken without exercise testing. For the non-exercise model, aerobic fitness is estimated from body mass index, self reported physical activity, age, and gender.

Body mass index (BMI) is calculated from weight and height. Self-reported physical activity is determined from Table 6.2, where you are asked to rate your level of physical activity for the previous 30 days on a 0 to 7 scale.

The procedures for estimating VO_2 max from the Non-Exercise Model are located in the Aerobic Fitness Lab Experience at the end of this module. Note that

once you estimate your physical activity level from Table 6.2 and your body mass index, you can use Table 6.3 (men) or Table 6.4 (women) to estimate your VO_2 max from the Non-Exercise Model.

EVALUATION OF VO$_2$ MAX

Standards for evaluation of aerobic fitness for males and females of various ages are presented in Table 6.5. The categories are divided into quintiles. The "low" category represents the lower 20% of the population and the "high" category represents the upper 20% of the population.

SUMMARY

Aerobic fitness is the ability to use oxygen to perform work. Adequate levels of aerobic fitness are important not only for sports performance, but also for health purposes. This chapter focused on aerobic fitness, but both aerobic and anaerobic exercises are important for overall health. Aerobic fitness can be estimated from several methods, including the PACER, Mile Run and the non-exercise model.

- Aerobic activities are those conducted continuously with large muscle groups in the presence of sufficient oxygen (e.g., walking, jogging, cycling).
- Anaerobic activities are usually of a high intensity so that sufficient oxygen is not available to meet the demand of the activity (e.g., weight lifting, running sprints).
- VO_2 max, also called maximal oxygen consumption, is the best index of aerobic fitness.
- VO_2 max is expressed relative to body weight as milliliters of oxygen per kilogram of body weight per minute ($mL \cdot kg^{-1} \cdot min^{-1}$).
- Several factors can influence one's level of VO_2 max, including age, heredity, gender, and current level of physical activity.
- The PACER and Mile Run are maximal tests of aerobic fitness. This means that maximal exertion is needed to perform these tests correctly.
- The non-exercise model can be used to provide an accurate estimate of aerobic fitness without exercise testing.
- The Healthy Fitness Zone represents a level of performance that provides some degree of protection from hypokinetic diseases and can be used to determine whether you have an adequate level of aerobic fitness or whether you need to improve your level of aerobic fitness.

TABLE 6.1

AEROBIC FITNESS TESTING

Name_____ Gender_____ Age ____

Height (feet and inches) _____ Weight (pounds) _____

MEN

Test	Healthy Fitness Zone	Your Score	Healthy Fitness Zone (Yes/No)
PACER (# laps)	≥ 44	_____	_____
Mile Run VO$_2$ max (mL·kg^{-1}·min^{-1})	≥ 44.3	_____	_____
Non-Exercise Model VO$_2$ max (mL·kg^{-1}·min^{-1})	≥ 44.3	_____	_____

WOMEN

Test	Healthy Fitness Zone	Your Score	Healthy Fitness Zone (Yes/No)
PACER (# laps)	≥ 38	_____	_____
Mile Run VO$_2$ max (mL·kg^{-1}·min^{-1})	≥ 38.6	_____	_____
Non-Exercise Model VO$_2$ max (mL·kg^{-1}·min^{-1})	> 38.6	_____	_____

FITNESS MATTERS: SUCCESS STORIES

WHAT STUDENTS SAY ABOUT THIS CLASS . . . .

This class helped by making me aware of my current health behaviors and how and why I should improve them. I really enjoy swimming now. — Brittany G.

I have begun cycling as a way to increase my aerobic fitness. — Alex B.

TABLE 6.2

CODE FOR PHYSICAL ACTIVITY*

Use the appropriate number (0 to 7) that best describes your general ACTIVITY LEVEL for the PREVIOUS MONTH.

Do not participate regularly in programmed recreation, sport, or heavy physical activity.

0 - Avoid walking or exertion, e.g., always use elevator, drive whenever possible instead of walking.

1 - Walk for pleasure, routinely use stairs, occasionally exercise sufficiently to cause heavy breathing or perspiration.

Participate regularly in recreation or work requiring modest physical activity, such as golf, horseback riding, calisthenics, gymnastics, table tennis, bowling, weight lifting, yard work.

2 - 10 to 60 minutes per week

3 - More than one hour per week

Participate regularly in heavy physical exercise, e.g., running or jogging, swimming, cycling, rowing, skipping rope, running in place, or engaging in vigorous aerobic activity type exercise such as tennis, basketball, or handball.

4 - Run fewer than one mile per week or spend fewer than 30 minutes per week in comparable physical activity.

5 - Run 1 to 5 miles per week or spend 30 to 60 minutes per week in comparable physical activity.

6 - Run 5 to 10 miles per week or spend 1 to 3 hours per week in comparable physical activity.

7 - Run more than 10 miles per week or spend more than 3 hours per week in comparable physical activity.

*Developed for use at NASA/Johnson Space Center, Houston, Texas.

TABLE 6.3

Estimated VO$_2$ Max (mL·kg^{-1}·min^{-1}) from the Non-exercise BMI Model for Men for Selected Ages and Body Mass Index Levels

Activity Level	Body Mass Index								
	16	18	20	22	24	26	28	30	32
Age 20 years									
7	61.1	59.6	58.1	56.6	55.1	53.6	52.1	50.6	49.0
6	59.2	57.7	56.2	54.7	53.2	51.7	50.1	48.6	47.1
5	57.3	55.8	54.3	52.7	51.2	49.7	48.2	46.7	45.2
4	55.4	53.8	52.3	50.8	49.3	47.8	46.3	44.8	43.3
3	53.4	51.9	50.4	48.9	47.4	45.9	44.4	42.9	41.4
2	51.5	50.0	48.5	47.0	45.5	44.0	42.5	41.0	39.4
1	49.6	48.1	46.6	45.1	43.6	42.0	40.5	39.0	37.5
0	47.7	46.2	44.7	43.1	41.6	40.1	38.6	37.1	35.6
Age 25 years									
7	59.2	57.7	56.2	54.7	53.2	51.7	50.2	48.7	47.1
6	57.3	55.8	54.3	52.8	51.3	49.7	48.2	46.7	45.2
5	55.4	53.9	52.4	50.8	49.3	47.8	46.3	44.8	43.3
4	53.4	51.9	50.4	48.9	47.4	45.9	44.4	42.9	41.4
3	51.5	50.0	48.5	47.0	45.5	44.0	42.5	41.0	39.5
2	49.6	48.1	46.6	45.1	43.6	42.1	40.6	39.0	37.5
1	47.7	46.2	44.7	43.2	41.7	40.1	38.6	37.1	35.6
0	45.8	44.3	42.7	41.2	39.7	38.2	36.7	35.2	33.7
Age 30 years									
7	57.3	55.8	54.3	52.8	51.3	49.8	48.3	46.7	45.2
6	55.4	53.9	52.4	50.9	49.4	47.8	46.3	44.8	43.3
5	53.5	52.0	50.4	48.9	47.4	45.9	44.4	42.9	41.4
4	51.5	50.0	48.5	47.0	45.5	44.0	42.5	41.0	39.5
3	49.6	48.1	46.6	45.1	43.6	42.1	40.6	39.1	37.6
2	47.7	46.2	44.7	43.2	41.7	40.2	38.7	37.1	35.6
1	45.8	44.3	42.8	41.3	39.7	38.2	36.7	35.2	33.7
0	43.9	42.3	40.8	39.3	37.8	36.3	34.8	33.3	31.8
Age 35 years									
7	55.4	53.9	52.4	50.9	49.4	47.9	46.4	44.8	43.3
6	53.5	52.0	50.5	49.0	47.4	45.9	44.4	42.9	41.4
5	51.6	50.0	48.5	47.0	45.5	44.0	42.5	41.0	39.5
4	49.6	48.1	46.6	45.1	43.6	42.1	40.6	39.1	37.6
3	47.7	46.2	44.7	43.2	41.7	40.2	38.7	37.2	35.7
2	45.8	44.3	42.8	41.3	39.8	38.3	36.7	35.2	33.7
1	43.9	42.4	40.9	39.3	37.8	36.3	34.8	33.3	31.8
0	42.0	40.4	38.9	37.4	35.9	34.4	32.9	31.4	29.9

TABLE 6.4

Estimated VO$_2$ Max (mL.kg-1.min-1) from the Non-exercise BMI Model for Women for Selected Ages and Body Mass Index Levels

Activity Level	Body Mass Index								
	16	18	20	22	24	26	28	30	32
Age 20 years									
7	50.1	48.6	47.1	45.6	44.1	42.6	41.1	39.6	49.0
6	48.2	46.7	45.2	43.7	42.2	40.7	39.2	37.7	47.1
5	46.3	44.8	43.3	41.8	40.3	38.8	37.3	35.8	45.2
4	44.4	42.9	41.4	39.9	38.4	36.9	35.4	33.9	43.3
3	42.4	41.0	39.4	37.9	36.4	34.9	33.4	31.9	41.4
2	40.5	39.0	37.5	36.0	34.5	33.0	31.5	30.0	39.4
1	38.6	37.1	35.6	34.1	32.6	31.1	29.6	28.1	37.5
0	36.7	35.2	33.7	32.2	30.7	29.2	27.7	26.2	35.6
Age 25 years									
7	48.2	46.7	45.2	43.7	42.2	40.7	39.2	37.7	47.1
6	46.3	44.8	43.3	41.8	40.3	38.8	37.3	35.8	45.2
5	44.4	42.9	41.4	39.9	38.4	36.9	35.4	33.9	43.3
4	42.5	41.0	39.4	38.0	36.5	35.0	33.5	32.0	41.4
3	40.5	39.0	37.5	36.0	34.5	33.0	31.5	30.0	39.5
2	38.6	37.1	35.6	34.1	32.6	31.1	29.6	28.1	37.5
1	36.7	35.2	33.7	32.2	30.7	29.2	27.7	26.2	35.6
0	34.8	33.3	31.8	30.3	28.8	27.3	25.8	24.3	33.7
Age 30 years									
7	46.3	44.8	43.3	41.8	40.3	38.8	37.3	35.7	45.2
6	44.4	42.9	41.4	39.9	38.4	36.9	35.4	33.8	43.3
5	42.5	41.0	39.5	38.0	36.5	35.0	33.5	31.9	41.4
4	40.6	39.1	37.6	36.1	34.6	33.1	31.6	30.0	39.5
3	38.6	37.1	35.6	34.1	32.6	31.1	29.6	28.0	37.6
2	36.7	35.2	33.7	32.2	30.7	29.2	27.7	26.1	35.6
1	34.8	33.3	31.8	30.3	28.8	27.3	25.8	24.2	33.7
0	32.9	31.4	29.9	28.4	26.9	25.4	23.9	22.3	31.8
Age 35 years									
7	44.4	42.9	41.4	39.9	38.4	36.9	35.4	33.8	43.3
6	42.5	41.0	39.5	38.0	36.5	35.0	33.5	31.9	41.4
5	40.6	39.1	37.6	36.1	34.6	33.1	31.6	30.0	39.5
4	38.7	37.2	35.7	34.2	32.7	31.2	29.7	28.1	37.6
3	36.7	35.2	33.7	32.2	30.7	29.2	27.7	26.1	35.7
2	34.8	33.3	31.8	30.3	28.8	27.3	25.8	24.2	33.7
1	32.9	31.4	29.9	28.4	26.9	25.4	23.9	22.3	31.8
0	31.0	29.5	28.0	26.5	25.0	23.5	22.0	20.4	29.9

MODULE SEVEN
BODY COMPOSITION

OBJECTIVES

- Understand the differences between body mass index (BMI) and percent body fat.
- Understand the importance of BMI in determining health risk status.

FITNESS MATTERS: SUCCESS STORIES

WHAT STUDENTS SAY ABOUT THIS CLASS . . . .

Learning about the health-related issues associated with overweight and obesity have made me realize I need to make changes in my lifestyle. — Emily H.

The overweight/obesity lecture impacted me because it is so easy to become overweight and it helped me see that there are a lot of things people can do to prevent this. — Adrienne A.

The Overweight/Obesity lecture put in perspective healthy weight rather than image. — Megan G.

Body Mass Index (BMI) is the most common method for determining weight-related health risk. BMI is calculated by dividing weight in kilograms by height in square meters. While this might be confusing at first, once you understand the numbers and how they relate to establishing weight-related risk, BMI can be a useful tool in helping you make healthy decisions regarding your body weight.

Limitations with BMI are: 1) it does not differentiate between fat and fat free mass and 2) it does not assess location of fat (waist vs. hips). It is possible for someone to have a high BMI due to excess muscle and not excess fat. This is called a "false positive." In this situation, it appears that the individual has a high level of body fat when he or she does not. False positives are often observed in athletes and body builders. Conversely, it is possible for someone to have a normal BMI and excess body

fat (false negative); this is often observed in older adults.

One way to avoid incorrectly classifying someone as being at risk for weight-related health problems is to determine his or her body composition (percent fat). Determination of percent fat can be done in a variety

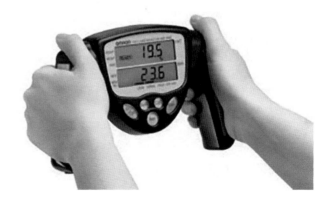

TABLE 7.1

Classification of BMI-related Disease Risk

	BMI (kg/m^2)	Health Risk
Underweight	< 18.5	Increased
Normal	18.5 – 24.9	
Overweight	25.0 – 29.9	*Increased
Obesity Class:		
I	30.0 – 34.9	*High
II	35.0 – 39.9	*Very High
III	40	*Extremely High

* Health risk relates to type 2 diabetes, hypertension, and cardiovascular disease.

of ways; one method commonly used to assess large groups quickly is bioelectrical impedance analysis (BIA). Your percent body fat will be determined by this method as part of the Physical Fitness Test you will take. To prepare for the BIA determination of your percent fat, see Module 3 for instructions. To get valid body composition results using this method, it is important to follow the assessment guidelines. This method relies on being well hydrated,;being dehydrated can result in an over prediction of your body fat level.

Additionally, you will calculate your BMI level, instructions for doing this procedure can be found in Module 2 of your text. When assessing health risk by BMI, it is important to understand that an optimal range of BMI exists, and once a person exceeds this range a corresponding increase in weight-related risk results. Table 7.1 provides the BMI levels and their associated health risks. Overweight is defined by BMI levels between 25 – 29.9 kg/m^2. Obesity is defined by BMI levels ≥ 30 kg/m^2. While weighing too much is associated with health problems, weighing too little (< 18.5 kg/m^2) is also associated with increased morbidity and mortality rates.

BMI is calculated with the following formula.

$$BMI = weight \ (kg) \div height^2 \ (m)$$

HEALTH RISKS ASSOCIATED WITH BMI

As previously mentioned, BMI is a sensitive indicator for establishing weight-related health risk in the majority of the adult population. When one's BMI is below (less than 18.5 kg/m^2) or above (more than 24.9 kg/m^2) the recommended ranges there is a corresponding increase in health risk. For individuals with BMI levels of 30+ range, health risk status changes much more dramatically. See Table 7.1.

Obesity is associated with increased risk for: cardiovascular disease, stroke, type 2 diabetes, kidney failure, orthopedic problems, cancer, depression, etc. As BMI levels rise above 35 kg/m^2 weight-related risk increases exponentially. A BMI of 35+ kg/m^2 is associated with a 600% increased risk of developing type 2 diabetes. When BMI levels exceed 45 kg/m^2 a loss of life expectancy is observed. However, a high BMI is not always associated with negative health consequences.

It is possible to have a high BMI due to increased levels of lean body mass (muscle) and not fat. Excess fat is typically associated with high BMI levels, although there is a subset of the population that has a high BMI which is due to having a large amount of muscle. Professional football players (Figure 7.1) can be misclassified as being at health risk when

FIGURE 7.1

Vonta Leach, a past East Carolina University Pirate standout, is an excellent example how BMI can inaccurately assess weight-related health risk.

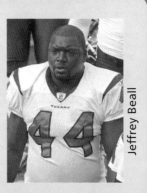

Jeffrey Beall

Vonta is six feet tall and weighs 246 pounds. His calculated BMI of 33.5 kg/m² places him in the obese category. In his 11 years in the pros, he has been to the Pro Bowl three times and has earned a Super Bowl ring. His 40-yard dash time is 4.87 seconds. It should be obvious by his success and athletic ability that his high BMI is due to muscle and not fat.

TABLE 7.2

Healthy Percent Fat Ranges Based on Age and Gender

STANDARD	AGE GROUP IN YEARS			
	Under 30	30 – 39	40 – 49	over 49
ADULT MEN				
High	> 28%	> 29%	> 30%	> 31%
Moderately High	22 – 28	23 – 29	24 – 30	25 – 31
Optimal Range	11 – 21	12 – 22	13 – 23	14 – 24
Low	6 – 10	7 – 11	8 – 12	9 – 13
Very Low	< 6%	< 7%	< 8%	< 9%
ADULT WOMEN				
High	> 32%	> 33%	> 34%	> 35%
Moderately High	26 – 32	27 – 33	28 – 34	29 – 35
Optimal Range	15 – 25	16 – 26	17 – 27	18 – 28
Low	12 – 14	13 – 15	14 – 16	15 – 17
Very Low	< 12%	< 13%	< 14%	< 15%

High — Percent fat at this level indicates that a person is seriously overweight to a degree that this can have adverse health consequences.

Moderately High — It is likely that the person is significantly overweight, but it could be due, in part, to measurement error. Based on risk factors and personal goals, weight loss and regular physical activity are recommended.

Optimal Range — It would be desirable to maintain body composition at this level.

Low — This would be a desirable body composition level, but further weight/fat loss should be discouraged. Fat levels that are too low are associated with negative health consequences.

Very Low — Percent fat levels at this level should only be reached by high-level endurance athletes who are in training. Extremely low levels might be due to measurement error. Fat levels in this range can be associated negative health consequences.

using BMI. When their body composition (percent fat) level is calculated a completely different picture emerges.

In a 2005 study in the *Journal of Strength and Conditioning Research*, body composition (percent fat) was determined on 53 members of the Indianapolis Colts' football team. Body composition was assessed using a technique known as air displacement plethysmmography (BodPod). This technique assesses body fat levels based on how much air is displaced by the subject in a fixed, volume container.

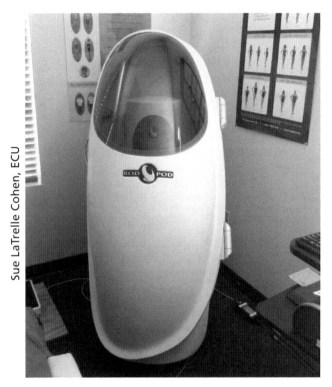

Sue LaTrelle Cohen, ECU

The body fat levels were assessed in 2003 at the end of the players' summer training camp. Athletes from all positions were assessed. BMI ranges were from 26 (kickers/punters) to 37 (offensive lineman). Based on BMI all athletes were at risk for weight-related health problems.

Body fat levels for the various positions ranged from 6.3% (defensive backs) to 25% (offensive lineman).

What this means is that an offensive lineman who weighs 308 pounds with 25% body fat will have a fat-free body mass (muscle, water, bone) of 231 pounds. These are explosive athletes that have the ability to get off the ball quickly and block defensive lineman.

This situation, though, is unique. To be this big and carry that much lean tissue requires an incredible commitment to fitness, very vigorous exercise training and genetics. Most people in the U.S. who weigh 308 pounds weigh that much because of excess fat, and not fat-free mass. In our lab, we have measured individuals with body fat levels in excess of 60%. For a 308-pound person this would mean 185 pounds of their body weight would be fat tissue!

While most of us are aware of the health risks associated with high BMI levels, what is not as well known and appreciated are the health risks associated with low BMI levels (< 18.5 kg/m^2). In the past several years France, Italy, Israel and Spain have passed new legislation banning models with BMI levels less than 18.5 kg/m^2 from fashion catwalks, photo shoots and advertising campaigns.

In comments by parliament members, the Israeli government blames the fashion industry for the widespread obsession with being skinny, because the "skinny obsession" places unreal expectations on young women while also creating body image issues and unhealthy practices necessary to maintain low BMI levels. Health risks associated with low BMI include: bone loss, decreased immune function, cardiac abnormalities, anemia and infertility.

In many cases the health risks associated with a low BMI result from not eating enough calories or an underlying health condition. When health conditions are controlled, low BMI levels can be attributed to eating disorders (bulimia, anorexia nervosa), excess exercise, smoking, drugs (diuretics, amphetamines) and other unhealthy behaviors.

PERCENT BODY FAT

Obesity is defined as having excess adipose (fat) tissue. The problem with BMI is that it does not differentiate between fat and fat free mass. It is possible to have a high BMI as a result of having a lot of muscle mass (false positive), as this is commonly observed in professional athletes.

Your body fat level will be determined by bioelectrical impedance analysis. To ensure a good estimate of your body fat level, you must adhere closely to the pretest instructions outlined in Module 2. If you have exercised within the previous 24 hours and/or are dehydrated, chances are that your body fat level will be overestimated.

As observed in table 7.2 body fat levels ranges change with age and sex. With age there is a loss of muscle mass. What this means is a person can carry the same body for their entire adult life and, due to biology, they lose muscle mass and gain fat mass. Thus their weight is the same but the proportion of fat and fat free mass has changed.

In addition to age-related reductions in muscle mass, women have approximately four times (12%) more essential fat than men (3%). Essential fat is necessary for maintaining normal biological functions. The extra essential fat levels for women help with fetal development and milk production.

SUMMARY

Weighing too much, or too little, is associated with the potential for developing weight-related health problems as assessed by BMI. The problem with BMI is that it does not differentiate between fat tissue and muscle tissue. Assessing percent fat provides more information relative to weight-related health risk status than BMI.

MODULE EIGHT

BASICS OF AEROBIC EXERCISE PRESCRIPTION

OBJECTIVES

- Understand the components of a safe and effective aerobic exercise prescription.

INTRODUCTION

In Module 5 we defined physical activity and exercise. Physical activity was defined as body movement that substantially increases energy expenditure. For most healthy and reasonably fit individuals, general increases in physical activity will enhance health, but dramatic changes in fitness or weight loss will probably not be seen. For those who wish to improve their fitness; a structured exercise program is needed with a focus on higher intensity, longer duration, greater frequency, and the type of aerobic exercise.

Developing a safe and effective exercise prescription depends upon knowledge of the components of a sound exercise program. In particular, the frequency, intensity, duration, and type of exercise should be considered. While most exercise prescriptions are primarily based on outcome-based goals (e.g., weight loss, improved fitness, health concerns), successful, long-term programs also need to focus on enjoyment. Your goals and interests will help you choose activities that are most appropriate for you. If you are interested in improving aerobic fitness and losing fat, aerobic exercise should be your priority. Weight lifting (a predominantly anaerobic exercise) is also helpful in obtaining and maintaining a healthy body composition. Resistance exercise

prescription will be addressed in Module 12. A well-rounded exercise program will generally include exercises that require both the aerobic and anaerobic exercise systems.

EXERCISE PRESCRIPTIONS FOR IMPROVING HEALTH AND FOR INCREASING AEROBIC FITNESS

Regular aerobic activity can increase aerobic fitness and improve your health. In this module, we highlight the exercise guidelines that are the foundation of a successful exercise program. Successful exercisers adhere to exercise guidelines developed by the American College of Sports Medicine (ACSM),the most respected institution in the world in terms of exercise. ACSM is the most

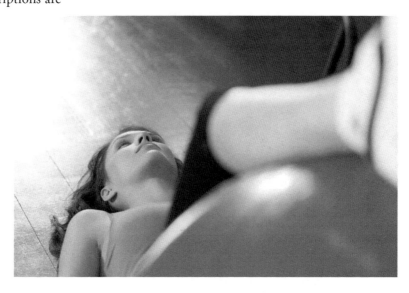

respected institution in the world in terms of exercise. The ACSM guidelines presented in Figure 8.1 are extremely important and useful.

Components of a sound exercise program include frequency, intensity, time, type, and enjoyment of exercise; also known by the acronym FITTE (Frequency, Intensity, Time, Type, and Enjoyment).

FREQUENCY

Frequency in the exercise prescription refers to the number of days per week. Based on numerous training studies, 3 to 5 days per week of aerobic exercise seems to be ideal for beginners. When beginning exercisers train for more than 5 days per week, the added improvement in VO_2 max is small. However, the injury rate associated with increased frequency of training above 5 days per week is substantial for beginners. Additionally, little or no changes in VO_2 max accrue with training regimens fewer than 3 days per week.

INTENSITY

Intensity refers to the level of the exertion, or how hard the workout is. Following are several methods commonly used to prescribe and monitor exercise intensity.

Heart Rate. A common way to monitor aerobic exercise intensity is through heart rate. Heart rate increases as exercise intensity increases. Because it is difficult to exercise at one specific heart rate and since the heart rate response to exercise varies from person to person, a range of heart rates is typically prescribed. This range of heart rates is termed the training heart rate zone. The lower limit of the training heart rate zone indicates the heart rate that would need to be reached in order for aerobic fitness to improve. The upper limit of the training heart rate zone minimizes exercise-related injury and promotes adherence. For beginners, highly intense activities are associated with injury risk, and lack of enjoyment.

> **KEY POINT**
> Determination of a training heart rate zone will provide you with a range of heart rates within which you should exercise to improve aerobic fitness and minimize risk of injury from activity that is too intense.

Rating of Perceived Exertion. Rating of perceived exertion (RPE) is another effective method to quantify exercise intensity. RPE is a measure of exertion used to gauge exercise intensity and for exercise testing and prescription. To use RPE, pay attention to how you feel during exercise and indicate your perceived exertion by assigning a number from the RPE scale to your feeling of exertion. RPE has

FIGURE 8.1

ACSM Guidelines for Developing and Maintaining Fitness in Healthy Adults

Frequency of training. 3 to 5 days per week.
Intensity of training. 50 to 85% of VO_2 reserve, or 50 to 85% of maximum heart rate reserve.
Time or duration of training. 20 to 60 minutes of continuous or intermittent [minimum of 10-minute bouts] aerobic activity accumulated throughout the day.
Type or mode of exercise. Any activity that uses large muscle groups, can be maintained continuously, and is rhythmical and aerobic in nature.
Resistance training. Strength training of a moderate intensity is recommended as an integral part of an adult fitness program. This aspect of fitness is discussed in the module on resistance training.

FIGURE 8.2

Rating of Perceived Exertion (RPE) Scale

0	Nothing at all
0.5	Very, very weak
1	Very weak
2	Weak
3	Moderate
4	Somewhat strong
5	Strong
6	
7	Very strong
8	
9	
10	Very, very strong
•	Maximal

If you are a beginning exerciser, use both heart rate and RPE to help maintain an appropriate exercise intensity. As you get a better feel for the relationship between heart rate and RPE, you can use RPE to gauge exercise intensity and heart rate can be measured less often. The use of RPE during an exercise session lets you monitor training intensity continuously throughout the entire workout. Additionally, as will be noted later, RPE can also be used to help you determine when it is time to modify exercise intensity. Many people do not monitor heart rate during exercise, but rather focus on RPE to gauge their intensity.

Intensity is the most difficult part of an exercise prescription. Intensity interacts with time, and to a lesser extent with frequency, and must be interpreted in context with duration of exercise. That is, intensity and time are inversely related. As the intensity of exercise increases, the time of exercise decreases. Simply put, you cannot maintain high-intensity exercise as long as lower intensity exercise. Importantly, this also means that as exercise intensity is reduced, you can exercise for a longer duration. The balance between these two components of an exercise prescription is important. Most people want to balance these two components in such a way that they can exercise at an intensity to improve their aerobic fitness, while at the same time exercise for a long enough time to expend a sufficient number of calories.

many cues; information from the cardiovascular system, the respiratory system, and working muscles is integrated to indicate a total, inner feeling of exertion. RPE should not be an indication of just one factor, such as leg fatigue or shortness of breath, but should be a feeling of overall exertion.

The modified **RPE Scale** ranges from 0 to 10 and is presented in Figure 8.2. Figure 8.3 indicates the relationship between oxygen consumption and RPE in the recommended training zone. In general, during aerobic exercise your RPE should be between 4 and 7.

TIME OR DURATION

Time refers to how many minutes you exercise per session. Because time of training interacts with intensity of training it must always be considered in

FIGURE 8.3

RPE Levels for Moderate to Very Hard Exercise Sessions

Intensity Level Category-Ratio RPE	%VO$_2$ max	RPE
Moderate	50 – 60	3 – 4
Moderate to Hard	60 – 80	5 – 6
Very Hard	85	7

concert with intensity. In general, exercise duration (exclusive of warm-up and cool down) can last from 15 to 60 minutes. However, a time of 20 to 30 minutes is appropriate for most individuals, especially for beginners.

Your exercise goals and what you find most enjoyable are important to consider when thinking about exercise intensity and duration. As long as you exercise above a minimal threshold (i.e., 50% of maximum heart rate reserve) for a sufficient duration, your exercise program will improve your aerobic fitness.

KEY POINT
Heart rate and rating of perceived exertion (RPE) are used to gauge exercise intensity. If exercise intensity is too high, it could lead to injury. If exercise intensity it too low, aerobic fitness gains may not accrue.

A program of low to moderate intensity, long duration exercise is typically recommended for beginners. This specifically relates to 40 to 60% of your heart rate reserve for a minimum of 30 minutes at least five times per week. This activity intensity will not provide the necessary stimulus for most individuals to make substantive exercise improvement; however, it will improve your overall health.

Depending on your fitness goals, you can vary the speed, duration and intensity to enhance your fitness results. While increasing intensity is the best way to improve fitness level, higher intensity exercise are associated with increased injury risk. It is possible to make fitness improvements by increasing duration or frequency of exercise and keeping the intensity constant.

TYPE OR MODE OF ACTIVITY

Many types of exercises can be aerobic in nature. To qualify as an aerobic activity it must involve large muscle groups, be rhythmic and be sustained for at least 20 minutes. An important point to consider when choosing the type of exercise you want to

perform is adherence. Whatever type of exercise you choose, it will only be beneficial if you actually do it. Therefore, choose activities that you find enjoyable.

Beginners or individuals prone to orthopedic injuries should choose mainly low-impact activities, such as walking, cycling, swimming, rowing, cross-country skiing, stair climbing machines, elliptical machines, and low-impact group fitness classes. High-impact activities include jogging, high-impact group fitness classes, basketball or other vigorous game activities, and jumping rope. These activities obviously place more stress on the joints and increase the rate of injury. Injury in the initial stages is one of the main reasons for dropping out of an exercise program. Therefore, beginning exercisers should do all they can to avoid injury.

ENJOYMENT OF ACTIVITY

Enjoyment means different things to different people. The idea of choosing activities that you like to do is easy to understand. Enjoyment of activity, however, can mean more than this. Enjoyment can also be thought of as a balance between the challenge the activity presents and your ability. People tend to find enjoyment in physical activities that meet or just exceed their abilities. For some, this may mean going for a bicycle ride on a trail that is just challenging enough for them. However, for others enjoyment may come in the form of CrossFit class or high-intensity indoor cycling class.

LIFESTYLE PHYSICAL ACTIVITY

To improve aerobic fitness, you must exercise at an intensity within your target zone. However, health-related benefits of physical activity can be achieved with lower intensity activities that characterize an active lifestyle (e.g., taking walks, gardening, cycling to work). Regular participation in lifestyle physical activities is an important adjunct to structured exercise programs.

SUMMARY

A realistic exercise program will help you meet your fitness and health goals. The components of frequency, intensity, time, type, and enjoyment of activity should be considered when developing an exercise prescription. Choosing activities that

FITNESS MATTERS: SUCCESS STORIES

WHAT STUDENTS SAY ABOUT THIS CLASS . . . .

I have learned how to properly do the exercises and can now create my own PA training program. I enjoy doing lunges and muscular strength training now. I also want to try more yoga. — Rachel K.

I learned more about the different equipment in the gym, which was helpful because I'm a freshman. Also, I learned about the different ways to exercise and enjoy it. — Ataya J.

By me taking this class and going through the motions in each concept, it allowed me to begin my weight loss program by using exercise from the activities. — Nicole E.

you enjoy or can learn to enjoy will help you stick with your exercise program. Heart rate and rating of perceived exertion (RPE) can be used to help monitor the intensity portion of the exercise prescription.

- The FITTE principle refers to the frequency, intensity, time, type, and enjoyment of exercise.

- Frequency of an exercise prescription refers to the number of days per week.

- Beginners should exercise 3 to 5 days per week. But remember to do some physical activity every day or nearly every day.

- Intensity is the most difficult part of the exercise prescription and is prescribed through heart rate or rating of perceived exertion.

- Exercise intensity and duration should be considered together and a balance must be reached to allow an exerciser to meet fitness goals.

KEY POINT

Many types of exercise can be used to improve your health and fitness, but none will work unless you actually exercise consistently. If you choose activities that you enjoy you are more likely to exercise consistently. Also, don't forget to add physical activity into your habits. A mistake new exercisers sometimes make is they look for ways to minimize spontaneous physical activity. This is called compensation. If you compensate by minimizing activity during your day because you now exercise, you lose out on an additional opportunity to enhance your health. So remember to take the stairs instead of the elevator, walk instead of ride, and go with your significant other for a walk rather than for a car ride.

MODULE NINE

SELF-MONITORING AND TECHNOLOGY

OBJECTIVES

- Understand how technology can be used to monitor physical activity.

INTRODUCTION

Students use a lot of different strategies to make lifestyle changes. One of the biggest predictors of success is s surprisingly simple—self-monitoring or tracking activity levels.

Self-monitoring is important because it helps you become more self-aware of how much, or how little, you do each day. Becoming more aware can help you recognize the need to change and also helps determine a realistic starting point in building an active lifestyle. Tracking your activity can also increase motivation. The simple act of recording tracking a mental routine that will help you stick to your exercise program. Tracking also helps you evaluate your progress. Sometimes actual physical changes are hard to notice as they are so gradual, but self-monitoring allows you to more easily see progress. Seeing progress is certainly gratifying, but tracking your behavior also lets you know when you are getting off track so you can make adjustments.

A variety of self-monitoring strategies exist, some of which are very simple and take little time to complete. For example, you could simply wear an activity tracker to monitor your activity level. Alternatively, you could record how much activity you did on an activity calendar

like the one shown on the next page. Others like to keep a training journal to track their activity and factors that affect motivation and performance. If you enjoy journaling, you might consider keeping an exercise log.

If you do not enjoy monitoring, then keep your monitoring system as simple as possible. If even that is too much, you could only self-monitor when you notice your physical activity levels are decreasing. The simple act of recording may prompt you to become more active.

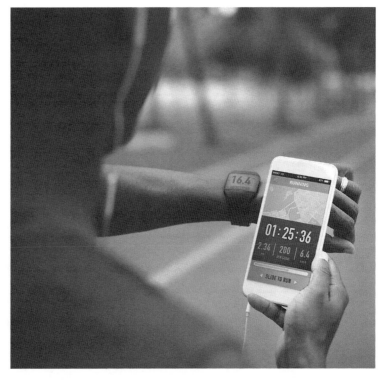

In recent years, technological advances like websites, apps, and wearable devices have made self-monitoring easy.

USING PEDOMETERS TO MONITOR PHYSICAL ACTIVITY

One way to monitor how active you are is by wearing an activity tracker. You may have heard that accumulating 10,000 steps per day is roughly equivalent to meeting 30 minutes of physical activity for health benefits. Why 10,000 steps? The average person walks close to 6,000 to 7,000 steps per day through activities of daily living. Thirty minutes of brisk walking accumulates approximately 3,000-4,000 steps. Adding 30 minutes of daily walking to normal lifestyle activity roughly then equals the 10,000 step goal for the average person.

People vary greatly in how many steps they take per day. Some people accumulate more than 6,000-7,000 steps per day while others may only get 2,000-3,000 steps per day. If you are currently not getting many steps, you might be meeting activity recommendations without reaching 10,000 steps if you are active for 30 minutes per day. Alternatively, you could focus on gradually increasing your step counts and challenging yourself to build up to the 10,000 step mark. If you are already walking close to 10,000 steps, you can get even greater benefits by adopting a more challenging goal than 10,000 steps per day or by increasing the pace at which you walk. One way to ensure you are walking at a brisk pace for health benefits is by walking at least 100 steps per minute.

KEY POINT

Americans can help stop weight gain by increasing physical activity and by decreasing caloric intake.

- Take 2,000 more steps per day (about a mile).
- Eat 100 fewer calories per day. Visit www.americaonthemove. org for more information.

Consuming 100 fewer calories a day is quite easy to do. For example, if you eliminate one 20 oz. soda a day you reduce your total caloric intake by approximately 250 calories each day.

TRACK YOUR STEPS CHART

Step Goal (baseline + 2,000 steps per day) = _____ steps per day

Day	Baseline Steps	Week 1	Week 2	Week 3	Week 4
Sunday					
Monday					
Tuesday					
Wednesday					
Thursday					
Friday					
Saturday					
Weekly Total					
Average Steps per Day					

Try some of these simple ways of building more steps into your day.

- Walk around when talking on your cell phone.
- Take stairs instead of the elevator whenever possible (it is usually possible whenever you are).
- Walk places instead of driving whenever you can.
- Park in a spot in the parking lot farther than you usually do, but be sure it is a safe parking lot when you do this.
- Take frequent walks. Short walks can add up to many steps.
- Walk your dog, even if you don't have one.
- Walk the mall in the mornings.

Other strategies to help you accumulate more steps each day are listed below. Remember that every little bit helps when burning calories.

- Get off the bus a stop before your usual stop and walk the rest of the way.
- Return the cart all the way into the store after shopping.
- Don't just stand there—move. Some people spend 10 minutes waiting for a bus. Instead walk up and down the sidewalk until the bus arrives.

- Rather than emailing or texting someone who is a short distance away, walk there and talk to them in person.
- When doing multiple errands, park in a central location and walk to your destinations.
- During TV commercials, actually get up and move.
- Play interactive video games instead of sedentary games.
- Don't use the drive through - park and walk to your destination (hopefully it's not a fast food joint).
- Take a 10-minute walk before or after lunch (or both).
- Join a walking group—the support might be just what you need.

APPS USED AS MOTIVATIONAL TOOLS FOR PHYSICAL ACTIVITY

Aside from pedometers and daily activity logs, technology has introduced various new innovative ways to help motivate you to be physically active and monitor your activity at the same time, simply by using your cell phone. Reasons people claim they do not exercise include: "I am too busy" or "I do not know what to do when exercising." Now many different phone applications are available that can help you get past the things that might keep you from being

FITNESS MATTERS: SUCCESS STORIES

WHAT STUDENTS SAY ABOUT THIS CLASS . . . .

I have recently downloaded the yoga app and have been doing yoga. — Jessica W.

Being introduced to mobile apps has been a huge help for me to track my exercise! I'm glad we were able to learn and use the apps in class! I love to run with an app I was introduced to in class! — Morgan B.

I tend to go running more often, and I enjoy using the Nike Running App. — DJ J.

Seeing how much I walk a day makes me want to walk even more. It is a personal trainer so-to-speak, on my hip. Hearing about obesity and all of the health conditions attached to it made me utilize every little bit of physical activity, including walking. I walk everywhere! I try to count my steps and then challenge myself the next day. — Katelyn C.

physically active. For example, when you are traveling, you typically take your phone with you. The ability to directly upload a workout to your mobile device has made exercising more convenient. Your phone can be used as motivational tools, but also they can also be used to monitor your physical activity levels. Some smart phone apps will record intensity of workouts and store all of your information in your profile. Research has shown that keeping daily logs of your activity and of what you eat can help you maintain or lose weight. Some popular apps are listed below:

Nike Plus App

This app is free. It allows you to map your runs using a GPS and set up a personal profile. In addition, this app allows you to:

- Track your progress throughout each run, including run time, pace, and calories burned.

- Keep a running diary by storing your information from previous runs, including the weather, the location in which you ran (outdoor vs. indoor), and the type of terrain (road, trails, or beach).

- Sync your activity with your choice of social media, including Facebook, Twitter, and Pinterest.

- Sync the app with your personal music playlist and include a "Power Song."

My Wellness Cloud

This is a free app that allows you to track all daily movement including physical activity, exercise and daily movement both done inside a recreation center, at home or outdoors. Daily MOVE goals are set for you based on your recent activity level; the goals adapt as your fitness adapts. Additionally, this app allows you to connect other devices and accounts to make tracking activity simple and concise. Accounts you can link to the MyWellness Cloud include:

- Fit Bit
- Garmin
- Map My Fitness
- My Fitness Pal
- Polar
- Run Keeper
- Strava
- Swimtag
- Withings

Swork It

The free app is built to work around anyone's schedule and allows users to adjust workout times to as little at 5 minutes. The workouts require no equipment and you can select from 20 pre-built workouts or create your own that focuses on cardio, strength, yoga or flexibility. Video instruction and audio cues are provided to take you through the workout and make it easy to follow along.

Yoga Studio

This app is available on Google play or through the iPhone App store. Yoga Studio allows you to have 24-hour access to a yoga classes that are provided through visual and audio instruction. The app includes 65 ready-made yoga classes with beginner, intermediate and advanced options as well as 15 minute, 30 minute or 60 minutes class times. You can choose to focus on strength, balance, flexibility, relaxation or a combination.

MyFitnessPal

This free app includes a food database to choose items you have eaten. In addition, this app allows you to:

- Keep track of everything you eat—a food diary and all of your exercise activity.

- Show your daily caloric intake and caloric expenditure.

- Make goals.

SUMMARY

New technology, like websites, apps, and activity monitors, can be used to help you self-monitor your physical activity levels and can provide motivation to keep you going. Using these services can complement your workout as well as your wallet because many are free. Search and enjoy trying a variety of new workouts.

- Pedometers are useful tools to determine present activity levels and to motivate people to be more active.

- Many apps are available to help you plan and monitor your exercise.

MODULE TEN

GOAL PLANNING

> **OBJECTIVES**
>
> - Understand the characteristics of effective goals
> - Demonstrate the ability to implement effective goal planning principles

In addition to self-monitoring, discussed in Module 9, effective goal planning can go a long way in helping you lead an active lifestyle. Students who set goals, develop a plan for how to achieve them, and monitor their progress are more likely to achieve success than those who do not. The scientific evidence is convincing: goal planning works. However, it is not enough to say "I want to get active and fit." Learning how to effectively use goal planning can help you achieve success.

Individuals with goals typically give more effort and persist longer in the face of obstacles than those without goals. Goals also provide a sense of purpose. Students who are striving to attain a goal are more likely to stick with physical activity compared to those who do not have a goal in mind. Without fitness or physical activity goals, it is easy to find reasons to skip workouts. Goals can help you experience a sense of accomplishment as you accomplish them and see performance improvements. That sense of success serves as a source of motivation. Finally, effective goals provide direction by focusing your attention on what you need to do in order to succeed.

We often find students have mixed feelings about goals. Some feel goal-planning works very well and is a key to success, while others are more ambivalent about how well it works for them personally.. a great deal of research has demonstrated that goals improve performance and motivation. However, research has also shown that goals do not automatically work. Certain types of goals are more effective than others. Oftentimes a reason why students have not experienced success with goal-planning is because they haven't implemented it effectively.

Before we discuss effective goal planning principles, list one or two physical activity and fitness goals you have for yourself. Then we'll go through and evaluate how well those goals meet effective goal characteristics.

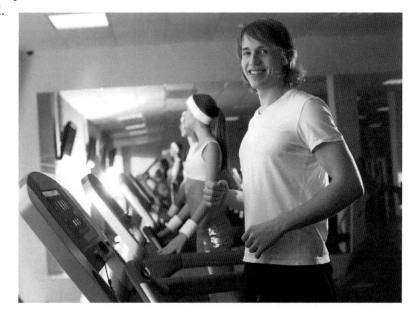

MY PERSONAL GOALS

1. _____
   _____
2. _____
   _____

SET SPECIFIC GOALS IN MEASURABLE TERMS

Specific goals stated in measurable terms are more effective than general goals. Specific, measurable goals can be quantified. They have a number attached to them. Statements like "my goal is to get fit" or "exercise more regularly" are too general. Neither of those goals is stated in specific and measurable terms. Specific goals might include, "my goal is to increase the number of steps I take per day this week by 1000," "my goal is to run a 5k road race in 21 minutes by the end of the summer."

Which of these goals is better? "My goal is to decrease caloric intake by 200" or "my goal is to drink one less soda per day." The second goal is better because it states specifically what the person will do. Although goals like "my goal is to swim three times a week for at least 30 minutes," or "my goal is to take three 10-minute walks on at least three days this week" are somewhat specific, they can be improved by making them even more specific. A more specific goal would specify on what days the person plans to exercise; otherwise, it is easy to put off exercise. You might even specify where, when, with whom to make the goal even more specific.

ACTION-ORIENTED

Many students are naturally drawn toward outcome or result-oriented goals. They say "I want to lose 20 pounds," "I want a flatter stomach" or "I want to bench press 250 pounds." In other words, they state an outcome or absolute endpoint they want to achieve. One problem with that approach is that these long-term goals might take an entire year, or even longer, to obtain. One solution is to have intermediate length goals. A person might state his or her goal is to lose 20 pounds in twelve months by losing 10 pounds in six months and 5 pounds in three months.

Although these increments are reasonable, there still is a problem with only having outcome goals. You can never guarantee that precise increments of change (weight loss, strength increase, running performance improvement…) will occur just because some physical activity program is followed for a given time period. Each person is unique and progresses at a different rate. Although the intermediate (e.g., three month) outcome goals might serve as a check to evaluate whether the physical activity program is having the desired impact, some people improve faster or somewhat slower than their stated goals. Outcome goals do not have to be set in stone; adjustments to your goals may be necessary.

Another important limitation of outcome goals, even short-term ones such as to lose 1 pound a week, is they do not focus on what you will do to achieve that goal. An effective solution is to include action-oriented goals. Action-oriented goals deal

---

K E Y   P O I N T

What is the key to lasting success and long-term success? SMART goals.

Specific	The goal specifies exactly what you are going to do or accomplish
Measurable	The goal can be quantified and progress can be measured
Action-oriented	The goal is associated with something you do and deals with <u>behaviors</u> that you will use to achieve desired outcomes
Realistic	The goal is achievable and within your reach
Time-Frame	The goal has a time frame and includes both long- and short-term goals

with specific physical activity or eating behaviors. These goals are called action goals because they are associated with something you do. For example, they might include doing 3 sets of 10 repetitions for each of the major muscle groups. Or action-oriented goals may specify running three times this week for 20 minutes coupled with walking an additional 20 minutes each time. In terms of eating, action-oriented goals focus on the types and amounts of foods. For example instead of eating cheeseburgers and fries 4 days/week they will opt for the baked chicken and sweet potato option.

There are two important advantages to action-oriented goals compared to outcome goals. First, you have more control over achieving action-oriented goals than outcome goals. Achieving action oriented goals is largely within your personal control and is determined by your effort.. Second, action-oriented goals create a path to achieving

desired outcomes. That is, to obtain desired outcomes, individuals need to change behaviors. The action-oriented goals provide the road map and daily guide for becoming more active. Action-oriented goals provide a sense of direction on how to achieve outcome goals by emphasizing the behaviors needed to obtain long term lifestyle change. Thus, action-oriented goals emphasize the behaviors you need to perform to achieve your long-term outcome goals.

One more thing about action-oriented goals, they should be positively rather than negatively stated. Negatively stated goals focus on what you want to avoid, positive goals focus on what you want to achieve. Rather than stating I'm going to stop eating junk food, state what you will do instead. The reason for positive goals is simple: it is easier to develop and build new habits than to break an old habit.

FITNESS MATTERS: SUCCESS STORIES

I got the job! In the fall I would be an EXSS 1000 instructor and teach students how to live a healthy life. After the initial excitement of getting the GA position, I was flooded with guilt and shame at my current fitness status. Little did I know that becoming an instructor would act as an antecedent to a lifestyle change that I hope to maintain for the rest of my life. On my first day of instructor training I had a BMI of 29.5 (obese is a BMI of 30 and above) and only completed 7 push-ups and barely reached 41 laps on the PACER. At 33% body fat, my 5'8" body frame did not look fit or healthy at 192 pounds. It was that day that I promised myself to change. I knew it would take time, but I was able to set small, manageable goals to help me reach my larger ones. First, I wanted to be consistently active. Running became my favorite form of physical activity because I could dissociate by listening to music and it was a great stress relief. After the first few months I began to switch up my workouts and started incorporating resistance training. I currently enjoy group fitness classes and interval training along with running. I also began monitoring my physical activity and food intake. Preparing healthy lunches for the week on Sunday nights helped prevent overeating and overspending. One of my best purchases was a Fitbit that I use to track steps, calorie expenditure, and daily mileage.

I was able to adhere to the plan I made for myself because I didn't cut out all of the foods I enjoy, made my exercise plan enjoyable and interesting, and I received so much support from my friends and family. Even my students began to notice a change in my appearance from the beginning of the semester! I don't always reach 10,000 steps each day, I still love chocolate, and push-ups will never be my favorite activity, but I will continue to improve and make strides towards a happier and healthier life. Oh! I can now do 62 laps on the PACER, complete 15 push-ups, and I'm down to about 25% body fat. And my 5'8" self now looks healthier at 162 pounds! (And I'm now in the healthy BMI range-24.5). — Autumn P.

A good strategy for setting action-oriented goals is to use the FITTE (frequency, intensity, time, type, enjoyment) principle that you learned about in earlier modules. To use the FITTE principle, you need to evaluate the strengths and weaknesses of your activity habits. What is your biggest weakness in terms of your activity program? Are you inactive too many days of the week? Do you need to build in longer workouts? Or do you need to increase your activity intensity? Then set a short-term goal to work on that component of the FITTE principle. In using the FITTE principle to set short-term goals, it is best to focus on one component of the FITTE principle at a time. For example, if you are running 30 minutes on three days a week, don't set the next goal to run 40 minutes on four days a week. A better goal might be to run 30 minutes on four days so only frequency is altered.

Action-oriented goals can also be used to increase enjoyment. If you are getting bored with your program, you can set a goal to try two new activities next week. If you like the social aspects of exercise, you can set a goal to call a friend to exercise for at least one of your workouts next week. You might set a goal to enjoy the scenery during a run. Setting good daily action-oriented goals should alleviate boredom because they give purpose and meaning to your workout.

REALISTIC BUT CHALLENGING

Ideally, goals should challenge a person but realistic enough to achiev If goals are so difficult that you seldom attain them, goals can lead to frustration and a sense of discouragement. At the same time, goals do not enhance motivation if they require no effort to achieve them. The key is to strike a balance between goal challenge and what you can achieve. As a general rule you should be at least 80% sure you can achieve your short-term goals, especially when you first start using goal-setting. You can always gradually increase the difficulty of your goals if you prefer to do so.

When first starting your journey to an active lifestyle, it is best to set goals that can be easily achieved and then gradually make the goals more difficult. You want to develop a solid foundation of success. When first using goal-setting, students sometimes start out with a lot of enthusiasm and excitement. Then after a few days, the whole goal-setting process seems like work and not too much fun. Setting goals that are

somewhat on the easy side and gradually increasing the difficulty can help prevent this. Remember, your ultimate reason for setting goals is to help you develop an interest in lifetime physical activity. Small, obtainable goals can help make an active lifestyle a reality. Also, setting too many goals can be overwhelming in the effort it takes to work on them. So, do not set too many goals at one time. One to three goals are ideal.

KEY POINT
Goal-setting Myth: Once you set a goal you have to keep increasing what you do each week by leaps and bounds. This is a myth. One reason people fail at goal-setting is they set the bar too high and find that working toward their goal is no fun. Unrealistic expectations about yourself and your goals can only hinder progress.

TIME FRAME: SET LONG-TERM AND SHORT-TERM GOALS

To make a commitment to your goals, place a time-frame or date on them. By when do you plan to accomplish them? In developing a time frame, realize that both long- and short-term goals are important. Long-term goals give you direction, but short-term goals get you to your destination Most people naturally set long-term goals that may take several months or even longer to obtain. Long-term goals are important - they are what you ultimately want to achieve. At the same time, long-term goals by themselves can be discouraging. Long-term goals may seem like they will never be obtained. Consequently, short-term daily and weekly goals are critical in enhancing motivation.

Short-term goals provide a sense of daily purpose. Many times improvements and progress toward long-term goals are so gradual that it is hard to notice improvements. Short-term goals help a person see progress and gradual improvement which may create a spiral of success. Attaining a short-term goal should result in feelings of success, which in turn lead to

FITNESS MATTERS: SUCCESS STORIES

WHAT STUDENTS SAY ABOUT THIS CLASS . . . .

It allowed me to focus on SMART goals to measure my improvement. Also, the lectures taught me about new machines and activities I find enjoyable so that I can have fun while I exercise. By having fun I am also more likely to achieve my goals. — Kirby G.

greater motivation, which should result in more success. In summary, both long-term and short-term goals are important, but short-term goals are critical in providing motivation on a daily basis.

One way to combine long-term and short-term goals is through the staircase approach to goal-planning. Think of a long-term goal as being at the top of the stairway and your current status at the bottom stair. Then include a sequence of progressively linked short-term goals connecting the bottom and top stairs. In using a staircase approach to goal-setting, it is important to make the steps small. You can think of each step in the staircase as being a "baby-step."

Goal Staircase

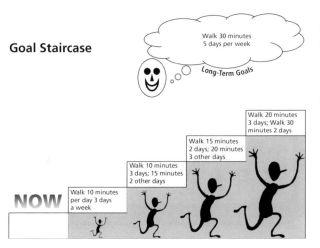

If you find you seldom obtain your short-term goals, you should consider making the steps smaller so you can obtain consistent success at achieving your short-term goals. For example, if you are currently sedentary, stating a goal to exercise 5 times a week for at least 30 minutes is a good long-term goal. An effective short-term goal might be to walk for two 15-minute bouts on Saturday, Tuesday, and Thursday and then gradually increase the number of minutes and pace you walk.

KEY POINT

Keep your long-term goals in mind but focus on your short-term goals. Start slow and gradually build up to long-term goals. Commit to a lifestyle change.

MY PERSONAL GOAL EVALUATION

Now let's go back and take a look at whether your personal goals meet the characteristics of effective goal-setting. Rate your personal goals on each of the characteristics of effective goal-setting by placing a check mark in the appropriate column if your goal conforms to that principle. If it does not, revise your goal to better meet the characteristics of effective goals.

Using the SMART goal approach can help you set effective goals, which can lead to a higher success rate in leading a healthy lifestyle. However, understanding SMART goals is not enough. We often see that students know how to describe SMART goals, but still struggle to accomplish their goals. This might be because they haven't implemented goal planning effectively.

KEY POINT

If we use effective goal planning, the process of working toward the goal is rewarding, not just achieving the end result. As stated in the cliché, "the joy is in the journey."

K E Y   P O I N T

Goal-Planning Myth: Once stated, goals should be set in stone. This is a myth. You need to continually set and revise goals, modify your action plan, and evaluate progress toward your goals. Goal planning is a flexible process and goals can be adjusted or revised at any time as life circumstances change.

AN EXAMPLE OF USING GOAL PLANNING

DeShawn decided that he wanted to increase his physical activity level. During the first week, he recorded his daily physical activity to establish a baseline. Following this, he set a goal of increasing his weekly workout time by 10%. He then set daily goals on how long he would like to workout each day and developed an action plan detailing strategies he would use to increase the amount he exercised. He then charted the amount he ran to see if his plan was working. Periodically, he monitored his running times to see if he was getting faster.

PERSONAL GOAL EVALUATION

	Specific/Measurable	Action-oriented	Realistic	Short-Term
Goal #1	_____	_____	_____	_____
Goal #2	_____	_____	_____	_____

Revised Goals:

_____

_____

_____

_____

_____

_____

_____

_____

MODULE ELEVEN
RESISTANCE TRAINING

OBJECTIVES

- Define the terms muscular strength and muscular endurance.
- Identify the benefits of resistance training.
- Understand the importance of spotting free weights.
- Identify common resistance training goals and common guidelines used to achieve these goals.

INTRODUCTION

In the previous modules we discussed goal setting and how this strategy could help you adopt healthy behaviors throughout your college years and beyond. One such healthy behavior is to add resistance exercise into a regular workout routine. This module will introduce you to resistance training concepts and definitions, the importance of muscular strength and endurance, common resistance exercises, and general resistance training techniques.

Muscular strength is the ability of a muscle, or group of muscles, to exert maximal force for a brief period of time. **Muscular endurance** is defined as the ability of a muscle, or group of muscles, to exert a submaximal force over an extended period of time. Adequate levels of both, especially as you age, are vital for performing activities of daily living (ADLs). In addition, both muscular strength and muscular endurance are essential to participating in common recreational and occupational activities, which are probably more interesting to you as a college student. Since you probably possess enough strength to perform ADLs, but a well-designed resistance training program aimed at improving muscular strength and endurance may improve your ability to participate in certain recreational activities,

such as playing basketball or hiking. Additionally, resistance training has been shown to improve body composition, improve body image, reduce risk of injury, and increase energy levels. Table 11.1 lists several benefits of including resistance training into your regular exercise routine.

SAFETY CONCERNS AND GENERAL RECOMMENDATIONS

Before we get into the technique used with specific lifts, we need to discuss some general guidelines to follow when performing resistance training exercises. The first thing is you must remember to breathe! This may sound silly, but when beginning resistance training many people forget the most important technique: breathing! During the **concentric phase**, or the shortening of the muscle or muscle group being used to perform the exercise, you

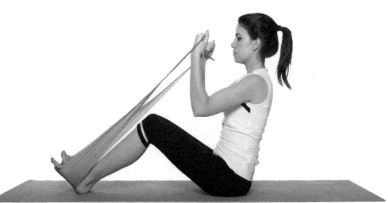

TABLE 11.1

Benefits of Regular Resistance Training

- Increased muscular strength and endurance
- Improved body composition
- Decreased risk of injury
- Improved self-image
- Improved posture
- Improved quality of life
- Decreased risk of developing osteoporosis
- Improved physical performance
- Improved self confidence
- Increased energy levels
- Improved health (for ex. regulate blood pressure)

East Carolina University Department of Kinesiology

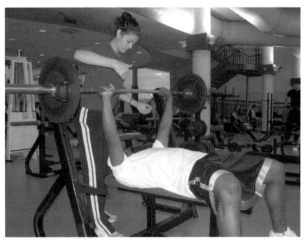

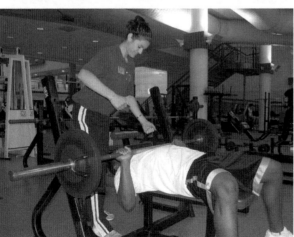

Figure 11.1: Barbell Bench Press with Spotter

want to exhale. During the **eccentric phase**, or the lengthening of the muscle or muscle group being used to perform the exercise, you want to inhale. An easier way to remember this breathing technique is to breathe out when the movement is more difficult and breathe in when the movement is easier. For example, when performing a squat the downward movement is the easier portion (eccentric phase) of the movement. Therefore, you should be inhaling during this phase of the exercise. The upward movement is the more difficult portion (concentric phase). In this phase of the exercise you should exhale. Failing to breathe during resistance training can result in dizziness, spikes in blood pressure, or even passing out.

When training with free weights (i.e., barbells and dumbbells) certain exercises should always be spotted to ensure the safety of the lifter. As a general rule, all exercises in which a barbell or dumbbell travels over the lifter's face or head while the lifter is seated or lying should be spotted. These exercises are some of the most dangerous to perform for fear of the weight collapsing on the head, face, or throat. An example of such lifts is the barbell bench press (Figure 11.1). During these lifts, communication between a spotter and lifter is essential. Before performing an exercise in which a spotter is needed, the spotter should know how many repetitions the lifter is aiming for and whether a lift off (assisting the lifter in unracking the barbell in the bench press) is necessary. If a lift off is needed, the lifter may say something like, "Ready on three. One, two, three." At this point the spotter should assist the lifter in unracking the barbell. The spotter should not release the barbell until the lifter has acknowledged that he or she has got it under control. During the execution of the exercise the spotter should remain attentive and ready to assist if the lifter shows signs of fatigue. After completing the exercise, the spotter should assist the lifter in re-racking the weight.

RESISTANCE TRAINING PROGRAM DESIGN

Your personal goals should be facilitated by your resistance training program. Whether your goal is to increase muscular strength, improve muscular endurance, or muscular hypertrophy (increase of muscle mass), there is a program for you! Sample workouts are provided in the appendices to this book to help you get started. When designing your

TABLE 11.2

Resistance Training Frequency Guidelines

Current Resistance Training Status	Frequency Recommendation
Beginner	2 – 3 days per week
Intermediate	3 – 4 days per week
Advanced	4+ days per week

personal resistance training program, you want to first think about training **frequency** or how many days you plan on training in a given week. Your training frequency will depend primarily on your current training status. Less experienced individuals will not require the same frequency as those with more experience. The primary reason is that less experienced individuals need more time (i.e., days) between resistance training sessions for their muscles to fully recover from the previous session. Table 11.2 provides you with frequency examples for individuals just beginning resistance training to those more advanced.

The **load** or amount of weight lifted and the number of **repetitions** performed are arguably the most important components when designing a resistance training program. Load and repetition assignments should be based upon the primary outcome goal of your overall program. The load and number of repetitions are negatively related in that as one goes up the other must go down. In Appendix 1, there are opportunities for you to test your 1-repetition max (1-RM) and/or repetition max (RM) for various lifts. If you choose to do these assessments, you can describe loads more objectively as percentages of a 1-RM or RM. For example, let's say you performed a 1-RM test for your back squat and worked up to 100 lbs for one repetition. You could then take a percentage of this load (i.e., 60%) and lift it for a prescribed number of reps (i.e., 8 reps). But for this lesson let's just describe loads using the following subjective terms: heavy; moderately heavy; and moderate. For your reference, a heavy load is one that can be lifted about 1 to 6 repetitions before fatigue occurs. A moderate load is one that can be handled for 12 to 20 repetitions. A **set** is defined as a group of

repetitions completed in a given sequence. The total number of repetitions (repetitions x sets) performed for a specific exercise can be referred to as the volume. For example, you may choose to back squat three sets of 8 repetitions at moderate load. This would equal a volume of 24 repetitions for the back squat.

FACT

Oftentimes, individuals will state that lack of time is the number one factor for not going to the gym. A well-designed resistance training program does not have to take a lot of time. By timing the amount of rest in between each set you can almost guarantee less than one hour in the gym, probably closer to 15 to 30 minutes.

The amount of time dedicated to recovery between sets is called a **rest period**. In general, as the load being lifted is increased so too will be the length of the rest period. Like load and repetition assignments, the assignment of sets to be performed and rest periods is dependent on the primary outcome goal, but also by your current training status. Less experienced individuals can perform fewer sets with longer rest periods and get the same benefits as long as the load and repetitions assignments are in place. Table 11.3 lists traditional assignments for loads, repetitions, sets, and rest periods based on one's primary goal.

TABLE 11.3

Guidelines to Resistance Training Programs Design According to Primary Goal

Primary Goal	Relative Load	Repetitions	Sets	Rest Periods
Muscular Strength	Heavy	1 – 6	2 – 6	2 - 5 minutes
Hypertrophy	Moderately Heavy	6 – 12	3 – 6	30 - 90 seconds
Muscular Endurance	Moderate	12 – 20	2 – 3	≤ 30 seconds

FACT

Weight Room Etiquette
1. Re-rack your weights after you are finished.
2. Wipe down equipment after you are finished.
3. In between sets be considerate of your fellow exercisers and allow individuals to "work in" with you while you rest.
4. If you move a piece of equipment after using it, please return it to its rightful place.

MYTH: If you stop lifting weights your muscle will turn to fat.

Just because scientists can turn sand into glass does not mean that your body can turn muscle into fat or vice versa. This myth probably stems from the fact that a lot of former athletes decrease their activity levels after they are finished competing, but do not decrease their caloric intake accordingly. This excess energy (extra calories) is stored as body fat.

MYTH: Women who weight train will develop big, bulky muscles.

No myth could be further from the truth and the proof is in the hormone testosterone. It is one of—if not the main—muscle-building hormone found in the body and is predominantly a male sex hormone. Women can produce testosterone, but generally produce 10 to 30% less than their male counterparts. Therefore, simply engaging in a resistance training program does not mean that a female will develop large muscles.

Another important factor influencing your program design is the **order** in which the exercises are to be performed. A general arrangement guideline to follow would be to perform exercises that use large muscle groups first (e.g., quadriceps, hamstrings, lattisimus dorsi, pectoralis major) followed by exercises that use smaller muscle groups (e.g., gastrocnemius, deltoids, biceps). Resistance training exercises are generally classified by the type of resistance they use and the number of joints involved. Single-joint movements such as an arm curl or a leg extension involve only one joint. Multi-joint movements like the back squat and pull-up involve two or more joints. As a rule of thumb, multi-joint movements should take priority (or be placed before) over single-joint movements because they will involve more than one muscle or muscle group and generally facilitate goals better than single-joint exercises.

FITNESS MATTERS: SUCCESS STORIES

WHAT STUDENTS SAY ABOUT THIS CLASS . . . .

Introduction to the weight room had the greatest impact on me because a lot of times when people go to the weight room, there is a sense of intimidation and not knowing where to start or how to use the machines. This day in class helped me get past that feeling. I find myself lifting free weights more often. — Julie B.

Both of the things I circled involve the weight room. I always wanted to learn more about the machines and how to use them. I also learned that it's okay for girls to lift weights! — Carson P.

So how do you decide which muscle groups to work during a given session? That is a great question and one that does not have a straightforward answer. A tried-and-true method is to perform lower-body exercises on one day followed by upper-body exercises on another day. So for example, if you are a beginner to resistance training you may want to perform lower-body exercises on Mondays and upper-body movements on Thursdays. For those more experienced with resistance training and currently training four days a week, a routine of lower-body exercise on Mondays followed by upper-body exercises on Tuesdays and repeat on

Thursday and Friday may be more appropriate. A routine like this will provide a greater frequency but still allow ample rest (at least 48 hours) for each body part.

SUMMARY

Incorporating resistance training can be a great complement to your regular workout routine. The guidelines in this module will assist you in developing a program to realize your goals. The benefits are numerous and many find resistance training very rewarding.

MODULE TWELVE
HEALTHY WEIGHT AND BODY COMPOSITION

INTRODUCTION

The addition of resistance training to a physical activity program can improve body composition by decreasing fat and increasing lean body mass. By assessing your body composition valuable information can be determined to help you determine your optimal, healthy weight.

HEALTH CONSEQUENCES OF OVERWEIGHT AND OBESITY

Overweight (BMI 25 – 29.9 kg/m^2) and obesity (BMI > 30 kg/m^2) are major health concerns in the United States and worldwide. According to the most recent BMI data for American adults: 31.2% were considered normal weight (BMI < 24.9) ; 33.1% were considered overweight (BMI 25 -29.) and 35.7% were identified has obese (BMI >30) . What this means is that 68.8% of American adults are at risk for developing weight related health problems. While the rate of obesity in the United States is slowing, obesity is considered a serious health problem. The health and social consequences related to obesity are numerous, have been well documented and include:

- Hypertension (high blood pressure)
- Elevated blood lipids (cholesterol, low density lipoproteins, triglycerides)
- Diabetes (type 2)

- Coronary heart disease
- Various cancers
- Congestive heart failure
- Stroke
- Gallstones
- Osteoarthritis
- Sleep apnea
- Cancer (colon, breast, endometrial, gallbladder)
- Lowered self-esteem
- Depression
- Substance abuse
- Employer discrimination (hiring prejudice, lower wages)

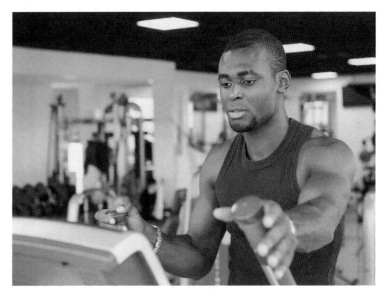

While this list is not complete, it should be obvious that obesity is, and will continue to be, a major health concern in the future. Perhaps more alarming than adult overweight and obesity rates are the rising rates for children and adolescents. Obese adolescents become obese adults, with the increasing rates of childhood obesity it is of no surprise that adult obesity rates have doubled since the early 1960s.

Decreases in physical activity and changes in dietary patterns appear to be primary causes of the obesity epidemic. In a short period (1900 to the present), our country has transitioned from an agrarian to an urban society. Technological advances have greatly reduced our physical activity patterns; jobs once done under "person power" are now performed with sophisticated machinery. Perhaps the largest impact on activity patterns has been America's love affair with the automobile. Seventy years ago most children were much more physically active. According to the father of one of the authors, who grew up in South Dakota during the great depression, he not only walked to school (two miles each way), but it was always uphill during a blinding snowstorm! What is becoming an area of increasing alarm is related to extended periods of sitting at the workplace. Sitting for hours at a time is associated with many health-related problems. In fact, if you do a quick internet search on the perils of sitting too much, you will find articles that compare the risk of sitting to be equal to that of smoking! A recent article found in the *Harvard Business Review*, "Sitting Is the Smoking of Our Generation," highlights this increasing health problem for YOUR generation! Clearly, inactivity is harmful to one's health, particularly for those who spend hours each day sitting at work or doing the Netflix binge.

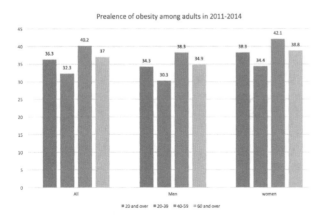

Figure 12.1 Adapted from CDC/NHS, National Health and Nutrition Examination Survey, 2011-2014

Changes in dietary patterns have also contributed to the obesity epidemic. The proliferation of fast food restaurants is frequently cited as a cause of obesity. During the period from 2007 to 2010, the Centers for Disease Control and Prevention (CDC) reported that approximately 11.3% of adult calories consumed were from fast food. The 20- to 39-year-old age group had the highest intake from fast food, averaging 15.3% of daily calories consumed.

The health consequences of excess weight have been well documented. A dose response relationship exists between BMI levels and mortality. As one's BMI increases above 24.9 kg/m², the risk of dying from heart disease increases quite dramatically. The most dramatic mortality rates are observed at BMI levels over 30 kg/m².

Excessive levels of obesity (Grade III, BMI ≥ 45 kg/m²) results in a quantifiable reduction in life expectancy. In a study that examined BMI and mortality, the authors reported a strong association between very high BMI levels and reduced life expectancy. Grade III obesity is associated with a reduced life expectancy of 12 to 20 years for Caucasian and African American males, respectively. Similarly, life expectancy was lowered by five years for Caucasian females and an average of eight years for African American females. Many studies have demonstrated that excess weight is strongly associated with increased morbidity and mortality rates from all causes (e.g., cardiovascular disease, cancers, stroke, accidents, suicide, etc.).

Although the relationship between reduced life expectancy and high BMI levels is well documented, weighing too little can also impact longevity. Levels below the recommended BMI range of 18.5–24.9 kg/m² result in increased mortality rates. While the reasons for this observed mortality risk are numerous, some deaths can be attributed to a lifestyle that promotes excessive dieting and risky health behaviors. The desire to be skinny is not a risk-free endeavor for some. Health risks associated with low BMI levels include premature bone loss, decreased immune function, cardiac abnormalities, and iron deficiency anemia.

While much is known regarding obesity and associated health risk, little has been written about the health risks of weighing too little (BMI < 18.5 kg/m²). The health consequences of low BMI levels were recently brought to light in the fashion industry following the death of a model with a BMI of 13.5 kg/m². As a result of the young woman's untimely death, organizers from the Madrid Fashion organization have banned models from their runways with BMI values less than 18 kg/m². Many health experts applauded this body weight restriction stating that it was long overdue.

Unfortunately, in many cultures, attractiveness is associated with being "model thin." Below are the heights, weights, and BMI levels of women who at one time or another have been popularized in the press as being beautiful women. While it is likely these women are healthy, only Megan and Victoria could walk the runway in Spain.

Name	Height (inches)	Weight (pounds)	BMI (kg/m²)
Taylor Swift	70	119	17
Kourtney Kardashian	60	116	17.11
Victoria Beckham	64	108	18.58
Megan Fox	66	114	18.4
Jessica Biel	68	108	16.4
Kate Beckinsale	68	115	17.5
Gabrielle Union	68	110	16.7

HEALTHY WEIGHT BASED ON CALCULATED BODY FAT

It should be clear that weighing too much or too little can be associated with negative health outcomes. For those of you concerned about your weight-related health risk, it is possible to compute your ideal weight. This can be easily done if you know your percent fat level. The assumption of the ideal weight prediction model is that there is an optimal fat range for individuals based on sex and age. This method does not evaluate health risks; it just provides a body weight range based on a predetermined healthy body fat level.

To determine ideal weight, percent fat level has to be determined. If you followed the instructions for having your percent fat determined by bioelectrical impedance in Module 3, then the calculation of ideal weight will be fairly accurate.

To calculate your ideal weight it is important to understand that ideal weight is based on the assumption that the weight loss ideally comes from fat mass vs. lean body mass. The best way to lose fat and maintain lean body mass is to combine caloric restriction with a regular exercise program that includes both aerobic and resistance training. Note that the calculation of ideal weight will not work if your weight-loss strategy consists of just caloric restriction. Losing weight without exercise results in the loss of both fat and lean body mass.

Your healthy weight range can be calculated based on your percent fat by using the steps below.

1. Determine fat mass: Fat mass = body weight * (%fat ÷ 100)

2. Determine lean body mass: Lean body mass = body weight – fat mass

3. Determine healthy weight: Healthy weight = Lean body mass ÷ (1 - healthy %fat ÷ 100)

FITNESS MATTERS: SUCCESS STORIES

WHAT STUDENTS SAY ABOUT THIS CLASS . . . .

Overweight lecture made me aware and opened my eyes to the path our country is leading down without classes like exercise. — Haley K.

It has affected me positively because I learned about how important it is to maintain a healthy weight. — Karsyn T.

Example: Calculate the healthy weight for a 25-year-old male who weighs 200 pounds and has 30% fat. The optimal range of percent fat for this person from Table 7.2 in Module 7 is 11-21% for a male under 30 years.

Fat mass = 200 x .30 = 60

Lean body mass = 200 - 60 = 140

Healthy weight (using range of 11% to 21%) = 140 ÷ (1 - .11) = 157 pounds

Healthy weight = 140 ÷ (1 - .21) = 177 pounds

In the above example, and depending on the desired fat level, our subject would need to lose between 23 (21%) and 43 (11%) pounds of body fat. If your body fat level or BMI level is too high, you might want to consider losing weight. However, before you decide to embark on a weight-loss program, you might first want to determine if you are at your healthy weight. Healthy weight should be based on your current weight, health, and recreational goals, therefore this varies for each individual. It is entirely possible to be overweight/obese by BMI and have excess adipose tissue as determined by % fat calculation and be considered healthy. The critical component in this equation is your aerobic fitness level. It is possible to be obese and aerobically fit. In this case being fit negates the health consequences typically associated with obesity.

REGIONAL FAT DISTRIBUTION

One last area to consider regarding adipose tissue is its location. Have you ever noticed wedding pictures of your parents? Fast forward 20-30 years and it would not be uncommon if both of your parents were 20-30 pounds heavier, and that your dad has gained the majority of his weight in the abdominal area and your mother has gained weight in the hip and thigh region.

Fat gained in the abdominal area is known as android obesity, and is characterized by an apple shape. Fat gained in the hips and thighs is termed gynoid obesity and is associated with a pear-like appearance. Excess fat that accumulates in the abdominal area is associated with a condition known as the "metabolic syndrome." This condition is characterized by a host of health problems, such as diabetes, high cholesterol, low high-density lipoproteins, high blood pressure, coronary heart disease, and certain cancers. A simple waist girth measurement is all that is needed to evaluate this condition. Waist girth is the smallest circumference between your lower rib and above the umbilicus. Men and women are at risk if their waist girth exceeds 40 and 34 inches, respectively. In contrast, gynoid fat distribution does not carry the same health risk.

SUMMARY

Obesity, determined by BMI and percent fat, is associated with premature mortality for men and women. Obesity rates have been linked to decreases in physical activity and increased caloric intake of energy dense foods typically found in fast food restaurants. However, recent studies have shown a strong relationship between aerobic fitness and decreased health risk status despite higher BMI and %fat levels. For individuals with a BMI in the 30-35 range that are aerobically fit, it appears that fitness, not fatness, predicts eventual health outcome.

For all of those who have been unsuccessful in maintaining long term weight loss, perhaps a new health intervention strategy is to focus on improving fitness level instead of spending time focusing on weight loss!

MODULE THIRTEEN

EXERCISE AND WEIGHT LOSS

OBJECTIVES

- Understand the impact exercise and physical activity have on weight loss and maintenance.
- Evaluate different strategies for losing weight.

INTRODUCTION

The purpose of this module is to provide you with some background regarding strategies for losing weight and maintaining weight loss. Making the decision to lose weight is a personal choice. Losing weight is challenging, keeping it off is even more so. To be successful you have to be ready to make significant lifestyle changes.

Of the many available weight-loss programs, some are better than others. As a consumer it is important to choose the program that is right for you. No consensus exists on the best program to follow. Most programs, if followed closely, will promote weight loss; it is the maintenance part of weight loss that is the most critical. Additionally, program safety is a major concern. For example, the Atkins program helps people lose weight and health risks associated with certain diseases can be improved. However, long-term adherence to this diet is difficult due to limited food choices.

The American College of Sports Medicine (ACSM) has extensively researched the area of weight loss. Researchers representing ACSM have published a comprehensive position statement regarding weight loss and weight regain. The authors concluded that significant amounts of aerobic activity, supplemented with resistance training, were necessary for weight loss/maintenance success.

Based on their position paper, ACSM recommends the following when choosing a weight-loss program:

- Choose the program that is "right" for you.

- Choose a program that is reasonable in terms of what you have to do to be successful and safe. Be wary of programs that make unrealistic claims about weight-loss success. It is unhealthy to lose more than a couple of pounds per week. In fact, long-term weight loss is associated with small amounts of weight lost over a long period. Programs that use expensive supplements are not only costly, but can also be hazardous to your health. If the program does not include physical activity as an important part of the weight-loss equation—avoid it. Physical activity is required for successful weight-loss maintenance.

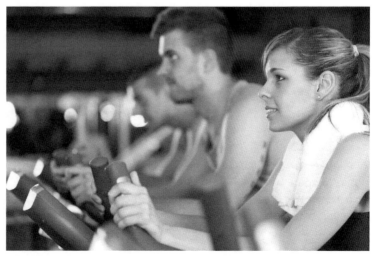

- Choose a program that is able to document long-term results. Losing weight is challenging, keeping it off is even more so.

[From: American College of Sports Medicine (2009). Appropriate Physical Activity Intervention Strategies for Weight Loss and Prevention of Weight Regain for Adults. *Medicine and Science in Sport and Exercise.*]

In addition to the above, ACSM recommends the following for weight loss programs:

- Initial weight-loss goal of 5-10% over a 3-6 month period.

- After the initial weight loss, work with professionals to develop maintenance strategies.

- Long-term success is directly related to modifying exercise and eating behaviors.

- Reduce energy intake by 500–1,000 calories per day, while focusing on keeping dietary fat intake below 30% of daily caloric intake.

- Progressively increase moderate physical activity to 150 minutes per week; extending exercise duration to more than 250 minutes per week is associated with long-term weight control.

- Include resistance training in your exercise program.

- Incorporate behavioral modification techniques.

EXERCISE, WEIGHT LOSS, AND MAINTENANCE

While the health benefits associated with physical activity and exercise have been firmly established, the amount of physical activity and exercise necessary to facilitate and maintain weight loss continues to be controversial. Some of the recommendations only focus on health, but are often misconstrued by the public as recommendations that facilitate weight loss. Weight loss/maintenance success is associated with longer duration aerobic exercise, supplemented by strength training, caloric restriction, and other lifestyle modifications.

Losing weight and keeping it off is not easy, but it can be done. A key to long-term success can be found from data generated from the National Weight Control Registry (http://www.nwcr.ws). The registry is the largest database in the world regarding common strategies necessary for successful weight loss and weight maintenance. More than 10,000 adults who have lost a

minimum of 40 pounds and maintained the weight loss for at least a year are included in the registry. For those of you interested in losing weight, here are some of the common success strategies used by registry participants:

- Eating breakfast.

- Frequent weighing, at least weekly.

- Watching less TV, the average participant watches less than 10 hours weekly (that's about one week of American Idol).

- Exercising at least 60 minutes per day.

In addition to exercise, it is necessary to reduce the number of calories consumed. While the formula for weight loss is simple, eating less and becoming more physically active is indeed challenging. It is not about drastically changing your diet, it is more about modifying behaviors that make you eat more and exercise less.

Understanding a little physiology may help you eat less. When full, our stomach sends a signal to our brain that lets us know we need to stop eating. However, there is a time delay from when the message from the stomach makes it to the brain. People who eat fast often eat more than necessary because of the time it takes for the feeling of fullness to reach the brain. To get that feeling of fullness (called satiety) before overeating here are some recommended eating strategies:

- 5-minute rule, wait 5 minutes before getting seconds.

- Put your fork down between bites.

- Chew food thoroughly.

- Talk during dinner, be engaged with your eating mates.

- Don't watch TV when eating, focus on the eating.

- Don't put serving dishes on the table.

- Use smaller dinner plates with similar proportions; when your plate looks full, your mind thinks, "wow, that is a lot of food, I won't be able to eat it all."

- Get up and move around after eating.

THE SKINNY ON EXERCISE AND WEIGHT LOSS

Numerous studies have evaluated the effectiveness of exercise on promoting and maintaining weight loss. Without a doubt, exercise is an important component; however, the ability of exercise to be the sole intervention strategy for weight loss is often misunderstood. Most people think that if they exercise they can eat anything they want. Unfortunately, that is not true. Exercise does expend calories, but the calories expended are much lower than most people realize.

Weight-loss success and weight maintenance depend on becoming more physically active. Creativity is important to become more physically active. There is a story about a woman who lived in a two-story house, and whenever she needed to use the bathroom she would always go to floor she wasn't on. Suppose this woman's extra stair activity resulted in her expending 10 extra calories each day. If she did this every day for one year, she would expend approximately 3,650 calories. This is the equivalent of losing one pound of fat.

One of the many misconceptions people have is about the power of exercise in promoting weight loss. While long-term weight-loss success is dependent on exercise, for the vast majority of our population it is not possible to use exercise as the only successful weight-loss strategy. It is possible to estimate the number of calories expended during exercise to illustrate this point. For those who exercise on equipment (treadmill, elliptical trainer, cycle), you know that if you enter your body weight you can see approximately how many calories you expend during exercise. Below is an example of how long it will take to burn off your favorite fast food meal with exercise.

This is an estimate and if you are using this as a guide and walking on a treadmill, the formula assumes you are not holding on to the rails and the treadmill is calibrated for speed.

Here's how it works.

"I was so hungry yesterday that I had to have a Hardee's Monster burger, large order of crispy curl fries, and a large sweet tea with unlimited refills." It doesn't take a rocket scientist to know that this is an unhealthy meal with a ton of calories, "but that doesn't worry me. I have the next day off so I'll spend some more time in the gym and work off the calories. Not a problem…."

A Monster Thickburger 2/3 pound (it was really good and I got it with everything) - 1,420 calories; crispy curl fries, large 5.4 ounces (I was really hungry) - 480 calories; sweet tea, 44 ounces (I was thirsty from the fries, burger, all the salt) - 600 calories.

Total for my really delicious meal = 2,500 calories.

So how long will I have to exercise the next day to burn all the calories from my meal (see example calculation below), at my current weight of 220 pounds? To burn off all 2,500 calories walking at a brisk 3.5 miles per hour pace, I would need to exercise for 6.5 hours (13 hours for someone who weighs 110 pounds)! While this is just an estimate, it does provide one with insight regarding how many calories are expended during exercise. Hopefully, this example makes it apparent that weight-loss success

FITNESS MATTERS: SUCCESS STORIES

WHAT STUDENTS SAY ABOUT THIS CLASS . . . .

As a result of this class, I got in contact with the instructor and they developed a workout/weight-loss plan for me. I will utilize this plan in an effort to lose weight and become a healthier person. — Kayla N.

By learning more about these concepts I was able to improve the way I exercise and manage weight loss, stress, etc. — Javier P.

I was introduced to ways that I could exercise without straining myself and without fear of passing out. I also understood the importance of weight loss and exercise. — Mandy C.

is dependent on physical activity/exercise, caloric restriction, and changes in eating patterns. When these behaviors are mastered, sustainable weight loss can occur.

For those of you interested in figuring out how long it would take to burn a given number of calories, simply fill in the blanks below (you'll need a calculator). The walking equation works for speeds between 1.8–3.8 miles per hour; use the jogging equation for speeds greater than or equal to 5 miles per hour. For speeds between 3.8–5.0 miles, the prediction equations do not work very well. If you happen to go that speed, then you can choose which equation works best for you.

Example Calculation for Walking:

1. The number of calories you want to expend? 2,500

2. Body weight in pounds? 220

3. Convert weight to kilograms (divide pounds by 2.2): 220 ÷ 2.2 = 100 kg

4. Pick a speed between 1.9-3.8 mph: 3.5

5. Multiply speed by 26.8. This converts mph to meters/min: 26.8 x 3.5 = 93.8

6. Take the value in number 5 above and multiply it by 0.10: 93.8 x 0.10 = 9.38

7. Add the value from number 6 above to 3.5: 3.5 + 9.38 = 12.88 (this represents the amount of oxygen your body needs each minute to walk at 3.5 mph)

8. Divide your weight in kilograms by 200: 100 ÷ 200 = 0.50

9. Now, multiply the value in number 8 above by the value in number 7 above: 12.88 x 0.50 = 6.44

This gives you the number of calories you would burn every minute. Now, divide the total calories of your meal by the number of calories you would burn per minute:

$$2,500 ÷ 6.44 = 388 \text{ minutes or } 6.5 \text{ hours}$$

This gives you the total number of minutes required to burn off the meal.

Example Calculation for Running:

1. How many calories?

2. Body weight in pounds?

3. Convert weight to kilograms: pounds ÷ 2.2 =

4. Pick a speed greater than 5 mph:

5. Multiply the speed by 26.8: 26.8 x mph =

6. Take the value in number 5 above and multiply it by 0.20:

7. Add the value from number 6 above to 3.5:

8. Divide your weight in kilograms by 200:

9. Now, multiply the value in number 8 above by the value in number 7 above:

This gives you the number of calories you would burn every minute. Now, divide the total calories of your meal by number of calories you would burn per minute:

This gives you the total number of minutes required to burn off the meal.

Spontaneous physical activity is an important adjunct to exercise, because a substantial increase in caloric expenditure can result. Taking the stairs instead of the elevator, walking to the store instead of driving, and walking instead of taking the bus to class are just a few ways to increase spontaneous physical activity and caloric expenditure.

Exercise is an important component for losing and maintaining weight loss. Most people who have lost weight and have been able to maintain their weight loss have a common denominator: exercise. Without involvement in a regular exercise program, long-term weight loss is much more challenging.

SUMMARY

Excess body weight is a major problem. Almost 70% of the adult population in the U.S. is at risk for weight-related health problems. The health and economic costs of overweight and obesity are enormous. Losing weight promotes health. The most effective programs include caloric restriction, aerobic and strength training activities, and behavioral strategies that promote better eating habits.

MODULE FOURTEEN

EXERCISE INTENSITY: HEART RATE AND RATING OF PERCEIVED EXERTION (RPE)

OBJECTIVES

- Understand how to monitor exercise intensity with heart rate and rating of perceived exertion.
- Provide opportunities for students to develop a personalized exercise prescription.

INTRODUCTION

Monitoring your exercise intensity is important when you participate in aerobic and strength training activities. We introduced the idea of using heart rate and rating of perceived exertion (RPE) to monitor your exercise intensity in Module 8. This module will provide details on how to determine if your exercise heart rate falls within the appropriate training heart rate zone.

You can monitor your aerobic exercise intensity through heart rate. In this module you will learn to determine a range of heart rates within which you should exercise to improve your fitness level. This is your training heart rate zone. If you exercise within your training heart rate zone, then your aerobic fitness should improve.

PERCENT OF MAXIMUM HEART RATE RESERVE MODEL

The percent of maximum heart rate reserve model is a widely used model to estimate an appropriate exercise heart rate for safe and effective workouts. Heart rate reserve is the difference between maximal heart rate and resting heart rate. Thus, to use the maximum heart rate reserve model, both maximal heart rate and resting heart rate must be known or estimated. Maximal heart rate is the highest heart rate that can be

achieved by an individual. Maximal heart rate is often estimated by 220 – age. Resting heart rate is your heart rate during resting conditions and is typically lowest in the morning before you get out of bed. Resting heart rate can be measured by palpating the radial or carotid artery as described on the next page.

Recommended exercise intensity ranges are between 40 and 60% of maximum heart rate reserve for moderate intensity and between 60 and 85% of maximum heart rate reserve for vigorous intensity physical activity. Steps to calculate training heart rate zone with the percent of maximum heart rate reserve model are presented in Figure 14.1. Exercising above your target heart rate zone should be done with caution. One reason why is because it is difficult to exercise above your heart rate zone long enough to develop fitness. Additionally, it can be unsafe and most people find it less enjoyable. However, interval training

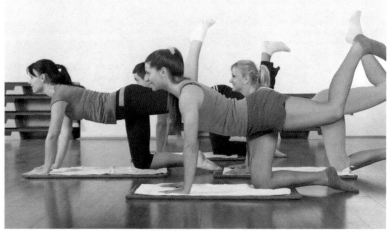

would be an exception in which case individuals intentionally train above their training heart rate zone.

Exercise heart rates between 60 and 85% of maximum heart rate reserve for various maximum heart rates and resting heart rates of 50, 60, and 70 beats per minute can be found in Table 14.1.

EXERCISE HEART RATE MEASUREMENT

In order to use heart rate to assess exercise intensity, you must be able to measure heart rate accurately. Heart rate monitors are now widely available and relatively inexpensive. Heart rate monitors fit snugly around the torso and transmit heart rate to a watch so that heart rate can easily be checked during exercise. Additionally, many smartphone apps have been developed to assess heart rate. By checking heart rate during exercise, you can immediately adjust your exercise intensity up or down depending on where your heart rate is relative to your training heart rate zone.

For people without a heart rate monitor or smartphone, exercise heart rate can be measured by palpating the pulse at the radial artery or the carotid artery. The radial artery can be found on the thumb side of the forearm near the wrist. The carotid artery can be found on the side of the neck.

To measure heart rate, press gently on the radial or carotid artery until the pulse can be felt. Pressing too forcefully on the carotid artery can result in a reflex lowering of the heart rate. On some people the radial artery is easier to pick up, but on others the carotid artery is easier to detect the heart rate.

If measuring heart rate immediately after the cessation of exercise, find the pulse as quickly as possible and then count the number of beats for 10 seconds. If you count the number of beats for 10 seconds, multiply this value by 6 to get beats per minute. Table 14.2 is provided to help you convert the 10-second count to beats per minute.

FIGURE 14.1

Maximum Heart Rate Reserve Model

Estimation of exercise heart rate for a 20-year-old subject (40 to 85% of maximum heart rate reserve).

Step 1. Estimate Maximum Heart Rate: Maximum Heart Rate = 220 – age.
Maximum Heart Rate = 220 – 20 = 200 beats per minute

Step 2. Measure Resting Heart Rate. e.g., resting heart rate = 60 beats per minute

Step 3. Subtract Resting Heart Rate from Maximum Heart Rate to get Heart Rate Reserve.
Heart Rate Reserve = 200 – 60 = 140

Step 4. Multiply Heart Rate Reserve by lower limit of training heart rate zone (e.g., 40%).
140 x .40 = 56

Step 5. Add Resting Heart Rate to this value.
56 + 60 = 116 beats per minute

Step 6. Multiply Heart Rate Reserve by upper limit of training heart rate zone (e.g., 85%).
140 x .85 = 119

Step 7. Add Resting Heart Rate to this value.
119 + 60 = 179 beats per minute

The training heart rate zone for a 20-year-old subject with a resting heart rate of 60 beats per minute using the percent of maximum heart rate reserve model is 151 to 179 beats per minute.

TABLE 14.1

Vigorous Exercise Heart Rates from the Maximum Heart Rate Reserve Model (65 to 80%)

Age	Maximum Heart Rate	Resting Heart Rate		
		50	60	70
18	202	149 – 172	152 – 174	156 – 176
19	201	148 – 171	152 – 173	155 – 175
20	200	148 – 170	151 – 172	155 – 174
21	199	147 – 169	150 – 171	154 – 173
22	198	146 – 168	150 – 170	153 – 172
23	197	146 – 168	149 – 170	153 – 172
24	196	145 – 167	148 – 169	152 – 171
25	195	144 – 166	148 – 168	151 – 170
26	194	144 – 165	147 – 167	151 – 169
27	193	143 – 164	146 – 166	150 – 168
28	192	142 – 164	146 – 166	149 – 168
29	191	142 – 163	145 – 165	149 – 167
30	190	141 – 162	145 – 164	148 – 166
31	189	140 – 161	144 – 163	147 – 165
32	188	140 – 160	143 – 162	147 – 164
33	187	139 – 160	143 – 162	146 – 164
34	186	138 – 159	142 – 161	145 – 163
35	185	138 – 158	141 – 160	145 – 162
36	184	137 – 157	141 – 159	144 – 161
37	183	136 – 156	140 – 158	143 – 160
38	182	136 – 156	139 – 158	143 – 160
39	181	135 – 155	139 – 157	142 – 159
40	180	135 – 154	138 – 156	142 – 158
41	179	134 – 153	137 – 155	141 – 157
42	178	133 – 152	137 – 154	140 – 156
43	177	133 – 152	136 – 154	140 – 156
44	176	132 – 151	135 – 153	139 – 155
45	175	131 – 150	135 – 152	138 – 154
46	174	131 – 149	134 – 151	138 – 153
47	173	130 – 148	133 – 150	137 – 152
48	172	129 – 148	133 – 150	136 – 152
49	171	129 – 147	132 – 149	136 – 151
50	170	128 – 146	132 – 148	135 – 150
51	169	127 – 145	131 – 147	134 – 149
52	168	127 – 144	130 – 146	134 – 148
53	167	126 – 144	130 – 146	133 – 148
54	166	125 – 143	129 – 145	132 – 147
55	165	125 – 142	128 – 144	132 – 146
56	164	124 – 141	128 – 143	131 – 145
57	163	123 – 140	127 – 142	130 – 144
58	162	123 – 140	126 – 142	130 – 144
59	161	122 – 139	126 – 141	129 – 143
60	160	122 – 138	125 – 140	129 – 142

Note: The lower value of the range is 65% of maximum heart rate reserve and the higher value of the range is 80% of maximum heart rate reserve.

FIGURE 14.2

Your Guide to Judging RPE

0–1	This is the feeling you get when sitting or doing something sedentary or when you get up and walk slowly across the room. Your breathing and heartrate are not elevated.
2	This is the feeling you might get when taking a leisurely walk outside. There is only a very slight, if any, feeling of fatigue and your breathing is comfortable. Carrying on a conversation is easy (unless walking with Kemble in which case you prefer not to talk).
3–4	This is the feeling you get when on a brisk walk. Your heartrate is elevated above normal and you become more aware that your breathing rate is elevated. At this pace, you can still carry on a conversation.
5–6	This is the feeling you get when you are running late and walking at a fast pace. Your breathing rate is somewhat deep. You can still carry on a conversation but your sentences may be getting shorter.
7–8	This is the feeling you get when you exercise vigorously. You can carry on a conversation, but you may not be speaking in full sentences.
9–10	This is the feeling you get with a very intense workout. You can still talk in short phrases but prefer not to talk much.

RATING OF PERCEIVED EXERTION

To use RPE, pay attention to how you feel during exercise and indicate your perceived exertion by assigning a number from the RPE scale to your feeling of exertion. RPE has many cues: information from the cardiovascular system, the respiratory system, and working muscles is integrated to indicate a total, inner feeling of exertion. RPE should not be an indication of just one factor, such as leg fatigue or shortness of breath, but should be a feeling of overall exertion. See Figure 14.2 for a guide on how to assess and use the RPE scale.

TABLE 14.2

Conversion Chart to Transform Heart Rate Counted for 10 Seconds to Beats per Minute

Beats/10 seconds	Beats/minute
15	90
16	96
17	102
18	108
19	104
20	120
21	126
22	132
23	138
24	144
25	150
26	156
27	162
28	168
29	174
30	180
31	186
32	192
33	198
34	204

THE TALK TEST

Physical activity intensity can be easily monitored with the talk test. If you are participating in light intensity activity (e.g. RPE 0-2), you will be able to sing a song during the activity. For moderate intensity activity (e.g. RPE 3-5), you will be able to hold a conversation, but not sing a song during the activity. If the intensity of a physical activity is vigorous for you (e.g. RPE 6-10), then you will not be able to hold a conversation during the activity.

SUMMARY

Intensity is the most difficult part of the exercise prescription and is monitored with heart rate or rating of perceived exertion. Monitoring the intensity of your exercise will take some practice, but will help you understand and appreciate what a safe and effective exercise intensity feels like.

FITNESS MATTERS:
SUCCESS STORIES

WHAT STUDENTS SAY ABOUT THIS CLASS . . . .

Each of the lectures gave me a background on a topic that had always had a huge "?" over it, and I felt like I couldn't participate in physical activity because I didn't have that understanding. These lectures made me feel comfortable with the activities throughout the course and I don't feel so uncomfortable about physical activities anymore. I've begun to participate in body weight workouts at home as well as aerobics. — Morghan C.

The concepts above have impacted me throughout the course because I have learned a lot about exercises that I wouldn't have tried outside the class. I am now less hesitant to try something new in my exercise routine. Before this class I only did cardio exercises, now I incorporate resistance bands into my routine. I went and bought them because of this class. — Jessica M.

EXERCISE AND STRESS MANAGEMENT

OBJECTIVES

- Develop awareness of the relationship between stress and health.
- Understand why exercise is an effective stress management tool.
- Learn how to use physical activity to reduce stress.

INTRODUCTION

In previous modules, you've learned how to develop a physical activity program to improve health and fitness. In this module, you will learn about exercise and stress. Is exercise an effective stress management tool? If it is, how much exercise is needed? Are some types of exercise more effective in reducing stress than others? Or is it possible that thinking of adding exercise to an already busy schedule creates more stress? Keep reading to find out the answers.

College can be an exciting and fulfilling period of your life. At the same time, college can undoubtedly be stressful and challenging. Stress producers come in the form of major life events as well as daily hassles. The college years are accompanied by a variety of major life events that can be stressful, including moving away from home, leaving old friends, making new friends, the excitement of new relationships, the pain of old relationships dissolving, adapting to a new living location, busy class schedules, finding a job, choosing a major, and making career choices. Added to this list of major life events are the countless number of irritating daily hassles that create stress. Waiting in slow lines, bad drivers, misplacing keys or other personal items, too many interruptions, unexpected company, too much to do with too little time to do it, insufficient sleep, bad weather, dealing with unrealistic professors, and annoying roommates can all be stressors.

Stress is one of the most common problems we face—it reduces our ability to stay well. Too much stress, especially when it is prolonged and not managed effectively, results in physical and mental health problems. In fact, stress is thought to be responsible in part for two-thirds of all doctor visits prompting some to believe that stress should carry a "health warning" much like other health damaging things. Medical researchers recognize that many diseases are psychosomatic in nature. **Psychosomatic diseases** involve the mind and body. These diseases are not "all in the mind." Rather it means that there is a mind-body connection influencing the onset, progression, and severity of the illness. Some estimates suggest that at least 85% of modern diseases may be psychosomatic.

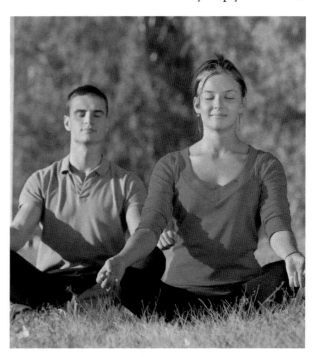

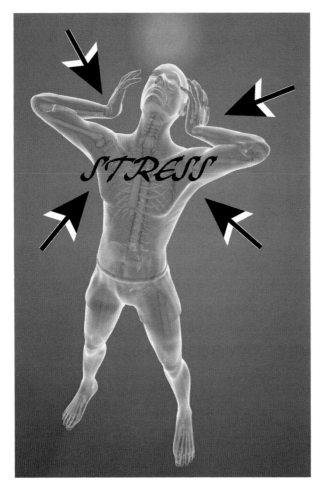

Figure 15.1

Chronic stress can impair your immune system and decrease your body's ability to fight off infectious disease and defend against illness. Any illness that is impacted by our immune system is influenced by stress. This includes a variety of illnesses ranging from minor respiratory infections and allergic reactions to more severe diseases such as cancer. Stress is also linked to coronary heart disease, stroke, high blood pressure, and arteriosclerosis/atherosclerosis. In addition, stress is associated with gastrointestinal difficulties such as diarrhea, constipation, heartburn, indigestion, irritable bowel syndrome, and pain associated with ulcers. Stress results in increased muscle tension, especially in the neck, shoulders, and back that can result in pain. Tension and migraine headaches are linked to stress. Stress can also affect blood sugar levels, which is potentially dangerous for a person with diabetes. Certain skin conditions like acne, hives, and herpes simplex are exacerbated by stress. Stress can be problematic for individuals with asthma. Stress also has a negative impact on male and female reproductive systems. No internal system is unaffected by stress and researchers are increasingly

recognizing that stress plays a role in the development, progression, and severity of many disease states.

Not only is chronic stress related to physical health problems, it is also associated with decreased mental health and reduced quality of life. Stress is linked to elevated anxiety, depression, anger, frustration, and most other negative mood states. Elevated stress is also related to lowered self-esteem and reduced quality of life. In addition, stress interferes with sleep, makes it difficult to concentrate, hinders decision-making skills, and impairs cognitive functioning. Stress can also create relationship difficulties. Individuals experiencing high stress can be impatient with others, irritable, short-tempered, and preoccupied with their self and personal needs.

Although the college years can be stressful, life does not automatically become less stressful after graduation. The reality is every life stage is characterized by its own unique sources of stress. After completing college you will experience a different set of stressors. In today's constantly changing world, most people find stress and pressure are the rule and not the exception. Given that stress is part of modern society, it is important to learn skills to deal effectively with stress. The habits you learn as a student, which include coping resources, can help you in life after college.

KEY POINT
Have you ever noticed during finals or when you are really busy that you get sick more often? This might be your body's response to stress.

COPING RESOURCES

Coping resources can be used to buffer the negative effects of stress. Three effective coping resources include good lifestyle management (e.g., healthy diet and sleep habits), social support, and exercise. Individuals with strong coping resources are less vulnerable to the negative effects of stress compared to those with inadequate coping resources. Strong coping resources provide stress resistance and bolster the ability to fight off stress-related illnesses. These resources can be thought of like a vaccine that helps protect a person from the negative effects of stress and enhance health.

Fitness helps buffer the impact of stress and thus staying active is a great coping resource. As shown in Figure 15.2, individuals experiencing fewer stressors (low stress) generally have fewer health problems than those reporting more stressors (high stress). This is true for both fit and unfit individuals. However, when experiencing a lot of stressors, fit individuals are at less risk of becoming ill compared to those who are less-fit. Thus, fitness offers protection against stress-related illnesses.

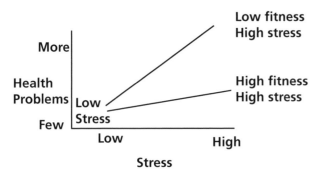

Figure 15.2

One of the reasons why fitness may help reduce the negative effects of stress is because fit individuals show a smaller physiological stress response than do less fit individuals (see Figure 15.2) and physiologically recover more quickly. When facing a stressor, fit individuals show a smaller increase in blood pressure, heart rate, and other indicators of a stress response and show a quicker return to normal levels. Because of this, regular exercisers may be less affected by stressors of daily living.

EXERCISE AND STRESS MANAGEMENT

Some research indicates that exercise may be as effective in managing stress as counseling techniques. Not yet convinced? College students rate exercise as one of the most common techniques they use to manage stress and also believe that exercise is one of the most effective techniques. Even a single workout can be a great stress reducer.

Exercise is effective at lowering stress levels for several reasons. After exercise, individuals show reduced sympathetic nervous system activity. Their heart rate and blood pressure are lowered. Exercise can relieve

TABLE 15.1

Exercise Guidelines for Stress Management

- **Frequency:** A minimum of three times a week to develop a fitness base for comfort. Whereas vigorous exercise can be performed 3 to 5 times a week, moderate intensity activity can be done on most, if not all, days of the week. Exercise needs to be regular enough so you feel comfortable while participating.

- **Intensity:** Both vigorous and moderate intensity exercise has benefits. The most important consideration is which intensity you prefer and enjoy. Some individuals do not enjoy high intensity exercise, whereas others find it enjoyable. Although intense exercise can reduce stress for some individuals, overtraining can negate the mental health benefits associated with exercise.

- **Time:** At least 20 to 60 minutes, but even short bouts (e.g., 10 minutes) have mood-enhancing and stress-reducing qualities. However, the mood-enhancing benefits are less pronounced and of decreased duration with short bouts of activity.

- **Type:** Activities that improve your mood and how you feel are optimal. Both aerobic and anaerobic activities are effective for reducing feelings of depression. However, aerobic activities often have larger anxiety-reducing qualities compared to strength training.

- **Enjoyment:** The most important consideration is to choose an activity that you enjoy. The ideal activities are ones that you find attention absorbing, provide a distraction from everyday life stress, or leave you with a sense of accomplishment.

muscle tension and also help metabolize the stress hormones underlying the stress response.

A good workout can also help minimize stress-producing thoughts and feelings. After exercising, students report feeling better. They may experience a sense of calm energy in which they feel relaxed and energized at the same time. Not only do positive mood states increase, negative feelings such as anxiety, depression, and anger decrease.

For some students, exercise provides a great time-out or distraction from stress. Others find that exercise helps them keep stress in better perspective and that they can think more clearly after a good workout.

Some students find it relaxing to let their mind wander during the workout, others experience a complete loss of thoughts if they get absorbed into the activity, and some find it meaningful to tune into their inner thoughts. Through exercise, people are able to envision new possibilities and solutions to problems that create stress.

Which types of exercise are most effective in managing stress? The good news is that the basic exercise guidelines for improving health provide a solid foundation for using exercise as a stress management technique (see Table 15.1). The most important consideration is to get active. Even a short walk can provide a distraction from stress and may

HOW DOES EXERCISE MAKE YOU FEEL?

You've learned in this module that exercise can be a great stress reducer and mood enhancer.

One of the most immediate benefits is that exercise can reduce stress and increase energy. The sense of feeling calm, but at the same time energized, following exercise might be a motivator for you. However, it is common to not feel like exercising. Sometimes people report "I just don't feel like exercising today" but then something happens. They go out and do some sort of physical activity. Afterwards they say, "I feel much better after I actually got out and walked." It is feelings like those that can help motivate you. Sometimes we are not fully aware of how exercise makes us feel. Because of that we encourage you to self-monitor your mood before and after exercise.

As a tool for self-reflection, you can use either the Feeling Scale or the Energy Scale presented below as a simple way to monitor your feeling states before and after exercising. You can record the information from these scales on your exercise calendar or exercise log.

Feeling Scale	*Energy Scale*
5 Very Good	6 Energetic
4	5
3 Good	4
2	3
1 Slightly Good	2
0 Neutral	1 Tired
-1 Slightly Bad	
-2	
-3 Bad	
-4	
-5 Very Bad	

help keep stress in perspective. More vigorous or longer duration exercise may provide added stress management benefits.

The best activities to help you cope with stress are ones that you enjoy, that you find attention absorbing, provide a distraction from everyday life worries, and that give you a sense of accomplishment. Some enjoy running, walking, or cycling because it gives them a chance to reflect and think. The rhythmical, repetitive movements can help quiet their mind as they get absorbed into the activity. Others may find those activities boring and prefer something like mountain bike riding or recreational sport if those activities are more enjoyable and attention absorbing. Some like working out with other people because of the social interaction and support. If you participate in an activity that you do not enjoy or find attention absorbing, it may actually create more stress. Finally, activities that provide a sense of accomplishment hold stress-reducing qualities.

Active individuals consistently report that exercise makes them feel better. However, the story is mixed when individuals are first starting an exercise program. Some mention that exercise improved their mood soon after they began their exercise program. Others mention that it took a few weeks for the feel-good sensations to develop.

So what is the bottom line? Most any type of exercise can be effective in managing stress. The key is to get up and move. When stressed, it is easy to forget about physical activity. However, keep in mind that being active can help you manage stress and deal effectively with challenging situations.

Another option for tracking your mood and exercise would be to use the form to the right. Each time before you exercise, take a moment and jot down your overall feeling at that moment. Then after you exercise, write down how you feel afterwards. It is important to select activities that help you not only feel better afterwards, but also while exercising. Even if you feel better afterwards, long-term motivation might be difficult if you feel bad during exercise.

Day 1

Before_____

During_____

After_____

Day 2

Before_____

During_____

After_____

Day 3

Before_____

During_____

After_____

Day 4

Before_____

During_____

After_____

FITNESS MATTERS: SUCCESS STORIES

WHAT STUDENTS SAY ABOUT THIS CLASS . . . .

Yoga was awesome. I loved how relaxing it was. I didn't know before I would like it. I already knew I enjoyed basketball but for the future I would like to do more yoga. — Jake M.

Yoga showed me an alternative way to exercise that also cleared my mind and helped with stress in general. — Haley K.

I am starting to do a little more yoga to be less stressed and more flexible. — Chris M.

What did you notice? Does exercise improve your mood and help you feel less stressed? Why do you think that might or might not be the case? Also, did you become aware of any specific activity types that are more effective in helping you feel better?

SUMMARY

Stress is part of our lives and needs to be managed. The reality is that every life stage is characterized by its own unique sources of stress. Fortunately, exercise can be a great stress reducer and mood enhancer. One of the most immediate benefits is that exercise can reduce stress and increase energy, even after one bout of exercise, so lace up your sneakers and go for a jog. While the benefits of exercise as a stress management technique have been well documented, it is possible trying to fit exercise into a hectic schedule can be stressful; therefore the positive effects of exercise might be diminished. It is important to choose an activity you enjoy and can easily fit into your schedule. Sometimes a simple 10 minute walk is all that is needed to clear your mind and relieve some stress.

STRENGTH TRAINING PRINCIPLES

OBJECTIVES

- Differentiate between one-repetition maximum (1-RM) and repetition maximum (RM) assessments for muscular strength.
- Be able to identify common principles associated with resistance training.
- Be able to apply more advanced concepts with various resistance training goals.

INTRODUCTION

In Module 12, we introduced you to the idea of resistance training for health-related fitness throughout adulthood and provided you with the basics to begin a resistance training program. In this module we will help you evaluate your muscular strength and endurance levels, provide you with principles that should guide your resistance training programs, and also give you some more advanced guidelines to follow if necessary.

Before beginning a resistance training program, it is important to determine your initial level of muscular strength and endurance. Muscular strength and endurance are specific to the muscle or group of muscles in question. Muscular strength may be expressed as: *absolute strength or relative strength.* Absolute strength is the total amount of weight that a person can lift or move. Relative strength is the total amount of weight that a person can lift or move divided by his or her own body weight (Relative Strength = Total weight lifted ÷ Body weight). The assessment of muscular strength and endurance can be done with relatively little time and/or money. Ways to assess muscular strength and endurance include:

- the one-repetition maximum (1-RM);
- the repetition maximum (RM); and
- tests utilizing body weight only.

Although most strength and conditioning specialists will agree that the 1-RM test is the "gold standard"

for assessing muscular strength, 1-RM testing is not generally recommended for individuals initially beginning a resistance training program. Therefore, these assessments will not be performed in class, but a description of each is provided in the Muscular Strength Appendix in the back of the text. We previously assessed your muscular strength and endurance using your body weight and you were able to compare your scores to those in the Healthy Fitness Zone (HFZ) in Modules 2 and 3.

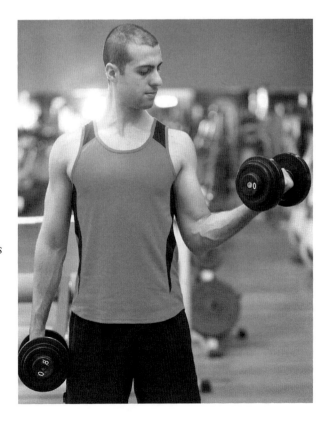

PRINCIPLES OF RESISTANCE TRAINING

In Module 12 we discussed information to help get you started in a resistance training program. Now we'd like to discuss four general training principles in regards to resistance training. However, please keep in mind these principles are part of all training programs, not just resistance training programs. The first principle of **specificity** refers to performing activities (i.e., lifts or exercises) that are specific to your goals. For example, if you wanted to increase the number of modified pull-ups you can perform in order to pass a health-related fitness test you may want to perform exercises such as bent-over or seated row, which work the muscles of the upper back (latissimus dorsi, teres major, trapezius, rhomboid, and posterior deltoid), which are needed to perform the modified pull-up. The principle of specificity can also be used interchangeably with the Specific Adaptations to Imposed Demands (**SAID**) principle. The premise of this principle is that the body will experience very unique adaptations based on the stress that is placed on it. For example, muscular strength will be better developed by incorporating heavier loads versus lighter loads.

The terms **overload** and **progression** have slightly different meanings, but for the purpose of this text we will combine them into one term, **progressive overload**. Progressive overload is a gradual and consistent increase in workload over time to ensure continuous gains are made. Progressive overload can be accomplished either by increasing the amount of weight or load being lifted, increasing the number of repetitions performed at a certain load, increasing the number of sets of a certain load and repetition prescription, decreasing the amount of recovery time or rest between sets, or simply by increasing the frequency of resistance training sessions.

If not applied correctly, progressive overload can lead to **overtraining**. During periods of overtraining, individuals can experience unusual fatigue and soreness and increased risk of injury. Therefore, it is common for strength and conditioning specialists to use the final principle of resistance training, **periodization**. Periodization is the systematic process of varying a training program at regular time intervals (e.g., every 4–6 weeks) to optimize gains in physical performance or other outcome goals. An example of periodization might incorporate four weeks of low-intensity, high-volume hypertrophy training followed by four weeks of high-intensity, low-volume strength training. While this principle was originally designed for highly skilled athletes, periodization can also help everyday exercisers avoid periods of overtraining and staleness in their resistance training programs.

MYTH: NO PAIN – NO GAIN!

You do not have to be sore after every bout of resistance training. In fact, most individuals would not continue resistance training if they were sore every day after training. Remember, lasting results do not happen in one training session. Results come from days, weeks, months, and years of a training regimen. So develop a program that you can adhere to for the long run!

MORE ADVANCED TECHNIQUES

In Module 12 we discussed some general recommendations and techniques used in resistance training. Now we will discuss some more advanced techniques that may be incorporated for additional progressive overload. The **speed of the contraction** is another important aspect of resistance training. It has been recommended that for every one second it takes to complete the concentric phase (shortening of the active musculature) of the lift, you should allow two seconds for the eccentric phase (lengthening of the active musculature) of the lift (1:2 ratio). However, this tempo does not hold true for all outcome goals, such as power or hypertrophy. Since the definition of power is force times velocity (or speed), the faster you move a given load the more power you will create. Please note while this is true, many facilities, including the weight room in the Student Recreation Center at ECU, discourage this type of lifting.

The term "**time under tension**" refers to the total amount of time a muscle or group of muscles is stressed during one set. This term is usually associated with hypertrophy training. Research shows that greater gains in hypertrophy are accomplished during the eccentric portion of a muscle contraction compared to the concentric portion. Therefore, a slower tempo (≥ 3 seconds of eccentric contraction for every 1 second of concentric contraction) would benefit those interested in gaining muscle mass. However, doing slower repetitions as described for hypertrophy will increase your dependency on a spotter. Additionally, performing slower eccentric contractions will increase **delayed onset muscle soreness** or **DOMS** (intense muscular fatigue and soreness that lasts several days after the lifting session has been completed). Therefore, for the purposes of this textbook, we recommend the 1:2 (concentric to eccentric) ratio. Or you can think of it as staying in control of the weight. You want to avoid "throwing" or "slamming" the weight. Always use smooth controlled movements and follow the breathing recommendations described in Module 12.

Since explosive lifting is not allowed in the Student Recreation Center, many college students will incorporate **plyometric training** into their fitness routine to increase power output. What is plyometric training? Plyometric training involves a rapid pre-stretch of the active musculature followed by powerful shortening of the same musculature. Let's examine the vertical jump for example. As an individual prepares to jump, he or she will first perform a countermovement (the quick pre-stretch of the quadriceps) before jumping as high as possible (the powerful shortening of the quadriceps). The benefits of plyometric training are two-fold. Obviously increased power output is expected. But additionally, athletes who engage in this type of training are less likely to be injured during sport compared to those who only train with slow movements. So if you wish to participate in intramurals or club sports, you may want to incorporate plyometrics into your training routine to not only improve performance, but also to reduce the risk of injury while competing. A sample plyometric training workout can be found in Appendix 2.

At various points throughout the semester, your teaching instructor may have led you through a day of **circuit training**. Circuit training is a useful way of incorporating various modes of training into one workout. For instance, one may perform push-ups, body weight squats, and jump rope sequentially with each exercise lasting for approximately 20–30 seconds (or for a specific number of repetitions) then repeat this process for the desired number of rounds. The benefits of circuit training include being a very time efficient workout that incorporates both muscular strength and cardio-respiratory rewards.

SUMMARY

In conclusion, your current level of muscular strength and endurance is important for goal setting and program design. Therefore, selecting a muscular strength test that best fits your goals and training status is key. When programming strength training into your overall workout routine, the principles of specificity (and SAID), progressive overload, periodization, and overtraining are important to consider. Finally, to insure long-term progression, there are several advanced resistance training prescriptions can be incorporated to get you through various plateaus or road blocks to your ultimate fitness goals.

FITNESS MATTERS: SUCCESS STORIES

WHAT STUDENTS SAY ABOUT THIS CLASS . . . .

I have become more comfortable going to the gym. I am now going to the gym 3 times a week, before this class I had never been to the gym before. — Jacob S.

I found that spending time in the weight room with the machines was beneficial by giving me exposure. I had used the machines in a gym at home, but visiting our gym on campus as a class helped. — Morgan B.

I learned some new techniques to use and now that I know how to use the machines I feel more inclined to go use them and not look like an idiot. I like core training! I do it at least 2 times a week now. — Ali C.

MODULE SEVENTEEN

ABCs OF BEHAVIOR CHANGE

OBJECTIVES

- Develop greater awareness of behavioral change tools you can use to achieve your physical activity goals.
- Learn how to apply the ABCs of behavior change to increase motivation.

INTRODUCTION

Success at leading an active lifestyle involves learning skills and strategies to become and stay active. You've developed some of these key skills in previous modules like self-monitoring and goal setting. In this module you will learn some additional behavioral strategies using the ABC's of behavior change that might help you achieve your health/fitness goals. When we ask students how they plan to achieve their goals, they often mention things like "I just need to be self-disciplined" or "I simply need to be motivated." Although strategies like that might work for a few days, they don't result in lasting change.

The reason why is simple—focusing on self-discipline, motivation, and willpower does not give direction on how to change or provide strategies that will help increase motivation. Rather than focusing on things like willpower, we emphasize "skill power" by providing tools that can help on the journey to an active lifestyle. Think skill rather than will.

The ABCs of Behavior Change

A ————————▶ B ————————▶ C

| Antecedents | Behavior | Consequences |
| (Prompts) | (Increase Activity) | (Reinforcers and Punishers) |

The ABCs of behavior change provide a useful framework for helping you achieve your goals. Previously,, we focused on tools to help you modify

behavior and increase your physical activity levels. The focus now is to learn skills that can be used to increase motivation by altering the antecedents and consequences associated with physical activity. This shifts the focus from willpower and self-discipline to changing one's personal environment to make activity more likely.

ANTECEDENT CONTROL STRATEGIES FOR BEHAVIOR CHANGE

Even though we may have good intentions to be active, we sometimes "slip" and go against our goals. We may simply feel that we missed a workout because we don't have enough motivation. If we look carefully we can often identify cues or antecedents that are the underlying cause. Antecedents are events that come before a certain behavior and trigger a person to act in a certain way. For example, feelings of hunger are an internal antecedent of eating. For some people, the time of day triggers eating; 5:30 may be an external

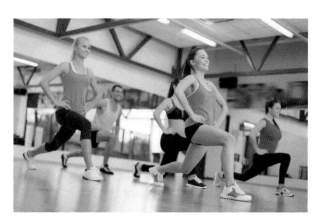

cue that triggers eating if a person eats regularly at 5:30. Coming home from school and seeing the remote may prompt TV watching. Similarly, many things can serve as a trigger or prompt for activity. Conversely, a variety of factors are antecedents that lead to inactivity.

The basic premise of antecedent control is to increase cues that lead to physical activity and decrease cues that lead to inactivity. For example, posting signs encouraging people to take the stairs, rather than the elevator, results in people taking the stairs. Why? The signs prompted or served as a cue to stair use. You can use the same types of strategies for yourself. Packing workout clothes the night before and posting reminder notes can help tip the scale in favor of working out. If the best time for you to exercise is after class, put your gym bag on the driver's seat of the car or wear your workout clothes to class. Scheduling exercise in your planner or calendar can trigger your being active. These simple actions serve as reminders to exercise and make it less likely you will skip your workout.

One student discovered that on the days he did not feel like working out he was more likely to exercise if he simply drove to the fitness center. Simply driving to the fitness center prompted him to go in and complete his workout. Conversely, another student noticed if she didn't feel like going for a planned run, she went for a walk instead. Oftentimes once she started the walk, she ended up running. If students are inactive, there might not be many naturally occurring cues prompting physical activity. Consequently, we need to develop cues that will eventually become associated with physical activity.

What cues can you use to trigger physical activity and meet your goals?

_____

_____

_____

_____

_____

In addition to increasing antecedents leading to activity, another strategy is to reduce the cues that trigger inactivity. These can be internal cues such as

feeling tired or stressed. They can also be external cues like the TV or couch. One student decided she would exercise at 5:30 p.m. each day before eating. However, when she came home, her roommates were typically watching TV. Although she had good intentions to work out, she often ended up watching TV instead. She also discovered that she was often hungry and did not feel like being active after a long day of school and work. The feelings of being hungry and tired resulted in her skipping her workout. To minimize the antecedents leading to inactivity, she decided to exercise before going home. Also, she noticed that if she ate a healthy lunch she was not as hungry at 5:30 p.m., which then made it more likely that she would exercise. Thus, she minimized the antecedents prompting inactivity.

What antecedents prompt you to be inactive?

_____

_____

_____

_____

_____

What strategies can you use to overcome those antecedents?

_____

_____

_____

_____

_____

WHAT ANTECEDENTS IMPACT YOUR ACTIVITY?

The key to making antecedent control strategies work is to discover what prompts or triggers you to be active and which cues make it less likely you will exercise. One way to discover the antecedents influencing your physical activity levels is through a physical activity log. On days you intended to be active, but were not, record the reasons why you were not. Then, on the days that you were active, note any special circumstance that led to your being active. By recording this information, you will develop insights into what makes physical activity participation more or less likely for you. Armed with that knowledge, you can be creative and design strategies to make physical activity easier by using antecedent control strategies.

USING SELF-TALK TO TRIGGER ACTIVITY

One often overlooked, but powerful antecedent, is your self-talk. Have you ever stopped and listened to how much self-talk is going on in your mind? If you are like many people, the little voice in the back of your head is constantly reminding you of what you should and should not do.

Applied to physical activity, students are often giving themselves instructions to either be active or to skip exercising. Some tell themselves negative instructions such as "I'm too tired to work out today." At other times, they rationalize their decision not to participate in activity, "I'll run after work rather than this morning" or "I want a clean start, so I'll start my exercise program on the first of the month." Although these excuses seem believable on the surface, on deeper inspection they are often unrealistic. Negative self-instructions and rationalizing make physical activity less likely.

Conversely, people who are successful at staying active use positive self-talk to motivate themselves. Positive self-talk guides students to achieving their goals. One might state, "I know I won't run if I wait until after supper. I'll just go for a light jog now" or "I'm tired, but I know I'll feel better when I'm done," or "It's a nice day, I will walk or ride my skateboard to class." Or you might say something even as simple as "three miles down, only one to go." When weight training, try "I know I can do this" or "just two more reps" when your mind is telling you to stop.

If you have a hard time maintaining an activity program, tune in to your self-talk by listening with a third ear to what the little voice in the back of your head is saying. If you notice that your inner dialogue is talking you out of being active, change the perspective you are taking and provide self-instructions that makes physical activity more likely. Just for practice, look at the box titled "Say What? Changing Self-Talk." Try to develop a positive self-instruction for each of the statements that will help you become active and break the thought chain.

MyThoughts+ is a great app to change negative self-talk. Every time you turn it on, it greets you with positive and affirming encouragement. You can also personalize your list with comments best suited for you, or create your own custom affirmations!

Antecedents or Cues to Action (or Inaction)

	Exercised	Did Not Exercise
Day 1		
Day 2		
Day 3		
Day 4		
Day 5		
Day 6		
Day 7		

SAY WHAT? CHANGING SELF-TALK

Negative Self-Instruction	Positive Self-Instruction
It's too cold outside, so I'll wait until a nicer day to walk.	
I want a clean start, so I'll start increasing activity on the first of the month.	

CONSEQUENCE CONTROL STRATEGIES FOR BEHAVIOR CHANGE

Consequences are events that come after the behavior and influence whether behavior is repeated. Consequences consist of reinforcements and punishments. Reinforcements include any consequence that increases the probability that you will repeat a certain behavior. Having fun, receiving recognition from others for being active, and the mood benefits associated with exercise are all potential reinforcers. They make it more likely a person will continue to be active. Any benefit a person receives from being active is a physical activity reinforcer.

Punishments include any consequence that decreases the probability you will repeat a certain

behavior. Some people experience several different "punishers" when they first start increasing their activity levels. They might comment that they dislike getting sweaty, do not like the feelings they have while exercising, and that they find the experience boring. In designing a lifetime fitness program, the goal is to maximize reinforcers and minimize punishments.

One reason why students may have a hard time is that they experience more punishers than reinforcers. Many of the natural reinforcers associated with an active lifestyle take time to develop. For example, students who are regularly active comment that they feel better and are less stressed when they are active. These are reinforcers for being active. However, in the first few weeks after starting to workout, those factors are not strong reinforcers because those benefits may not be readily noticeable. At the same time, numerous small punishers may be present. When first starting, students may not like the feelings associated with exercise, they may find the experience boring, and they may feel uncomfortable with how they look while being active. In developing a physical activity plan, it is important to decrease the punishers and increase the reinforcers associated with physical activity.

One strategy to minimize physical activity punishers is to lower the exercise intensity and focus on increasing lifestyle activity when first starting. Participating in intense exercise can be discouraging and painful if you have been inactive for a while. So if you are just beginning an exercise program it is

Adherence is increased if the scale is tipped in favor of reinforcers outweighing punishers

Punishers
Too time consuming
Too tiring
Dislike feelings while exercising
Boring
Feel uncomfortable
Feel awkward

Reinforcers
Look better
Feel better
Increased confidence
Increased energy
Improved health
External rewards

probably a good idea to start with moderately intense physical activity that feels good to you, rather than highly intense activity that feels overly hard on your body.

Another strategy to minimize the negative feelings is to change your attentional focus while exercising. While exercising, people can either cognitively associate or dissociate. Association occurs when individuals "tune in" to what their body is feeling and internal sensations such as heart rate, breathing, and how their muscles feel. Competitive endurance athletes often use association to monitor pace and as part of their race strategy. Association is also important in monitoring exercise intensity to make sure you stay within your target heart rate zone during aerobic exercise or to evaluate your RPE. However, many individuals benefit from dissociation, especially when they are first starting a program.

Dissociation occurs when a person tunes out sensory feedback. In dissociating, individuals may watch TV, listen to music, or talk to others to distract themselves from how they feel. They may also focus on the external environment, such as the scenery, or they may begin to daydream. Dissociation can make physical activity more enjoyable. Dissociation can reduce boredom and fatigue and help a person tune out some of the negative sensations he or she experienced during exercise. It can help overcome some of those immediate punishers you may have experienced when first beginning an activity program.

Along with reducing immediate punishers, another strategy involves increasing reinforcers by making exercise more rewarding. Striving for a reward can give you a boost of motivation and a proud feeling of accomplishment once you receive the reward. Knowing there is a reward waiting for us at the end of the line can be a powerful motivator and help us achieve higher and reach further.

For some students, being active is very intrinsically rewarding. Intrinsic rewards come from inside. These include the feelings of self-satisfaction you have for accomplishing personal goals or when realizing what your body can accomplish. Knowing you are doing something good for yourself and the positive feelings you may get from being active are also powerful intrinsic rewards. You may simply enjoy the feelings you have when being active, such as when you get absorbed in a sport game or workout. Intrinsic

rewards are undoubtedly one of the important motivators for being active.

Nothing can take place of those intrinsic motivators, but it takes time for activity to become intrinsically motivating for some. When first starting, it helps to build in extrinsic reinforcers or rewards. Have you ever noticed how some people initially go to 5K road races to receive a T-shirt? Receiving a T-shirt was an external reinforcer or reward that helped develop their interest in running. Eventually, the T-shirt becomes less important and they enjoy running for the sake of running. Before physical activity is part of an individual's lifestyle, extrinsic rewards can be used to help increase physical activity motivation. Over time, extrinsic rewards can be gradually faded out, as being physically active becomes part of one's self-identity and lifestyle. Extrinsic rewards might help focus your effort and give that extra shot of motivation to keep you going when you just do not feel like you can take that extra step. Extrinsic rewards can also serve as a gentle reminder to congratulate ourselves for a job well done.

Fitness clubs often use incentive programs and rewards to motivate members. You can also use rewards on your own to help increase your motivation. A variety of things can be used to reinforce physical activity. The chart on Characteristics of Effective Rewards includes some tips that might give you some ideas on what to use for a reward.

A critical part of the behavior change process is to develop greater self-awareness. This means becoming more acutely aware of your activity levels, but also aware of things that influence your activity levels, including antecedents and consequences. Without self-awareness you might not realize why you are, or are not, motivated, and what impacts your motivation. We cannot change what we are unaware of and many people overestimate their own self-awareness. Consequently, we encourage you to continue self-monitoring by keeping an exercise log, writing in an exercise journal, or even self-reflecting to help you develop greater self-awareness.

Increasing commitment to being active is also important. If being active is not important to you, all the tools discussed in this module will not be effective. To increase your commitment to an active lifestyle, we encourage you to continue to set goals (Module 10) and review the module on "What's In

CHARACTERISTICS OF EFFECTIVE REWARDS

- Rewards can be as simple as a gold star on your logbook each day or week you achieve your goal. One of the best reinforcers is feeling successful and simple rewards can be used to symbolize that success.

- Rewards must be valued. They can consist of material goods such as putting a dollar in a jar each time you exercise and then purchasing something you had your eye on, like a new outfit or sport equipment. Activities such as going to the beach or some other event can also be used to reward physical activity participation.

- The reward must be contingent on performing the desired behavior (physical activity) and not otherwise available. In other words, the person will not receive the reinforcer unless he or she meets his or her daily or weekly activity goal. Choose rewards that are personally valued, but that you will not take unless you perform the desired behavior.

- Rewards must move people toward their goals and not away from it. A trip to the ice cream store is not a good idea if a long-term goal is to lose weight. Rewards that promote even greater physical activity are ideal (e.g., new workout clothes, exercise equipment).

IDENTIFYING REWARDS

When using rewards, it's important to reinforce daily and weekly goal attainment rather than just long-term goals.

What are some ways you can reward yourself for achieving your short-term goals, such as your accomplishments today or this week?

_____
_____
_____
_____
_____

Now think big. Write down ideas for rewards that might help spur you on to reaching your long-term goal.

_____
_____
_____
_____
_____

It for You?" (Module 4) in which you evaluated the pros and cons of becoming more active. Focusing on your goals and the benefits of an active lifestyle can rekindle your motivation.

One additional way to increase commitment and use the ABCs of behavior change is to create a contract with yourself. Some students benefit from sharing their contract or plan with friends or family to further increase their commitment. Once you have put your commitment in writing and made it public, chances are you will take it seriously. Making your contract public may sound silly, but getting family and friends involved can go a long way toward motivating us when the going gets tough! Maybe share your goals on social media and ask your friends and family to hold you accountable.

KEY POINT
Putting your commitment in writing will help you take it seriously.

The sample contract on the previous page contains several features that make it a good one. First, it includes the target goal. It also specifies some strategies the person will use to obtain the goal. If you look closely, you will notice those strategies involve modifying antecedents. Finally, it includes reinforcements for achieving daily and weekly goals.

SAMPLE PHYSICAL ACTIVITY CONTRACT

Goal: To run a 5K road race

Time Frame: By June 10, 2014

To reach my goal, my weekly goals include:

- I will jog at least three days a week between my 11:00 and 1:00 class
- I will walk on at least two other days per week

Strategies to Achieve Goals

1. Carry my running shoes to school with me
2. Find a jogging partner
3. On the days I plan to walk, don't watch TV until after I walk
4. Schedule exercise time into my weekly planner

Rewards for Reaching Short- and Long-Term Goals

1. Reward myself with 30 minutes on the Internet each time I meet my daily activity goal
2. Take a trip to the beach if I meet my weekly goals for four weeks
3. Buy a new pair of running shoes after achieving my long-term goal

Overcoming Roadblocks

1. On rainy days, I will go to the recreation center
2. Exam days: I will jog after completing the exam to help clear my mind

Signed _____

Note: This contract will be revised on a weekly basis.

SUMMARY

Throughout this module, we focused on several tools using the ABC's of behavior change that provide students skills they can use to increase motivation to become or stay physically active. Although the ABCs of behavior change provide effective tools for helping students on their way to lifelong physical activity participation, those strategies only work if a person is (a) self-aware and (b) committed to becoming more active.

FITNESS MATTERS: SUCCESS STORIES

WHAT STUDENTS SAY ABOUT THIS CLASS . . . .

They made me realize the importance of healthy living, not just so I feel better about myself, but because I deserve to be healthy and treat my body right. I also learned a lot of new ways to exercise that are fun and enjoyable to me. — Landry V.

I didn't know much about PA or fitness before this class. These things helped me to have the knowledge and confidence to be more active, both at home and in a public setting. — Kailey A.

ADVANCED EXERCISE PRESCRIPTION

OBJECTIVES

- Understand how the components of an exercise prescription can be used to allow progression to even greater levels of fitness and health.
- Understand the three stages of an exercise prescription.

INTRODUCTION

Some of you started an exercise program at the beginning of this semester and progressed at an appropriate level with few issues such as soreness and/or injuries, but others of you may have progressed too quickly and suffered negative consequences. A successful exercise prescription should include consideration of progression and the initial, improvement, and maintenance stages of prescription.

PROGRESSION

Progression refers to the increase in exercise requirements as fitness improves. Exercise requirements can be increased by changing the frequency, intensity, and/or duration of exercise. The quickness with which you progress depends on a number of factors, among them are your age, health status, injury status, initial level of fitness, and fitness goals. Generally, older adult, diseased, overweight, and unfit individuals progress more slowly than others. Emphasis should be placed on beginning and progressing at appropriate levels. Do not start out with exercise that feels too strenuous or feel that you have to progress quickly. Your exercise prescription is individualized and the rate of progression should also be individualized.

Starting an exercise program with exercise that is too strenuous (i.e., too high of an intensity, too long of a duration, or too great of a frequency) can lead

to orthopedic injuries and/or dissatisfaction with exercise. Individuals who are injured early in an exercise program tend to discontinue their exercise program or are unable to progress as rapidly as they would have liked to if they were not injured. Beginning exercisers should not be overly concerned about intensity.

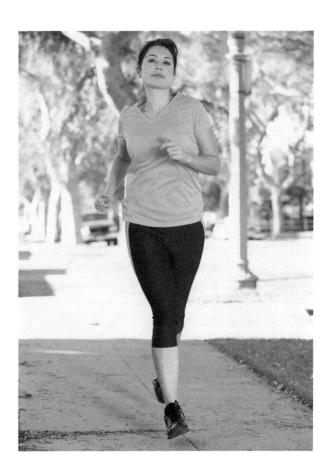

FITNESS MATTERS: SUCCESS STORIES

WHAT STUDENTS SAY ABOUT THIS CLASS . . . .

I learned something from each of the concepts that I know now, and will use in my everyday life. I now attend the gym 3 times a week. — Yameer G.

I have developed new, fun workout routines and regimens. I feel more confident in my physical activity limits and abilities. — Joy T.

People begin exercise programs for different reasons, but one thing is always constant, you must make a commitment to stick with it. Exercise for an adequate duration should be a short-term goal. Meeting goals can help you maintain your commitment. To review goal setting and goal planning principles refer back to Module 10. For beginners it takes some time (about three months for most people) before the pleasures of appropriate regular exercise are appreciated. It is important to get past this initial stage of exercise training with minimal soreness, few injuries, and a sense of enjoyment.

The need for progression can be judged based on your training heart rate and rating of perceived exertion (RPE). These concepts were covered in detail in Module 14. As you become more physically fit with training, your heart rate and RPE response to exercise will lessen. When your heart rate falls below the target heart rate zone, exercise intensity will need to be increased to maintain heart rate in this zone. When RPE during exercise falls below the target range [4 to 7 for the RPE scale], this is also an indication that exercise intensity can be increased.

Fitness goals also influence progression of an exercise program. If an increase in aerobic fitness is your goal, you should gradually increase exercise intensity to approximately 75 to 80% of heart rate reserve, duration to at least 30 minutes per session, and frequency to 4 to 5 days per week. A different exercise prescription could be used to meet the goal of a decrease in heart disease risk. Improvements in health can occur at a lower effort, such as an intensity of about 70% of heart rate reserve, duration of 30 minutes per session, and frequency of 3 days per week.

STAGES OF EXERCISE PRESCRIPTION

Generally, the prescription for aerobic exercise follows three stages: initial conditioning stage, improvement stage, and maintenance stage. Most beginners should start at the initial conditioning stage, but if you have already been relatively active and have an above average level of fitness you may choose to start at the improvement stage.

The initial conditioning stage should include moderate intensity aerobic activities (40–60% of heart rate reserve). The initial duration of the aerobic workout may only be 15 minutes, but is gradually increased as the activity feels comfortable. The main point of this stage is to get moving. The initial conditioning stage typically lasts for four to six weeks with a slow progression.

In the improvement stage intensity is gradually increased to the higher portions of the target levels (50–85% of heart rate reserve). The goal of the improvement stage is to improve fitness to the desired levels. This stage can last from 4 to 8 months. The maintenance stage begins after you reach satisfactory levels of fitness or after you reach some other predetermined exercise goal. If you were already in good condition when you began to exercise more regularly you may reach this stage sooner than if you were less conditioned. At the maintenance stage, intensity and duration may be held constant to maintain fitness. The goal of the maintenance stage is long-term maintenance of fitness levels. It is often a good idea to substitute various other activities to keep your exercise program interesting and enjoyable.

SUMMARY

The basics of a sound exercise prescription include the components of frequency, intensity, time, type, and enjoyment of physical activity. After you make fitness gains, you may want to consider how to change your exercise prescription to continue to improve your level of fitness.

- Progression in an exercise prescription refers to increasing exercise requirements as fitness improves.

- The three stages of an exercise prescription include the initial conditioning stage, improvement stage, and maintenance stage.

CARDIOVASCULAR DISEASE RISK FACTORS

OBJECTIVES

- Identify risk factors for heart disease.
- Understand the impact of regular physical activity on cardiovascular disease risk and mortality.
- Define heart disease.

INTRODUCTION

Module 19 focused on the basics of a comprehensive exercise prescription to help you continue to improve your level of fitness. What if you are improving your fitness level, but you smoke or are overweight, have high blood pressure, or have other health issues? Should you be concerned? This module explores the risk factors associated with cardiovascular disease.

WHAT IS CARDIOVASCULAR DISEASE (CVD)?

First and foremost, CVD is the primary cause of premature death for American men and women. Unfortunately, almost one out of two adults will die from this disease. While this might sound ominous, the good news is that for many, this is a very preventable disease.

The most common form of CVD is atherosclerosis. This disease is characterized by the formation of a waxy substance, known as plaque, within the arteries that supply the heart with blood. Over time, the plaque deposits grow in size, limiting the amount of blood that can get to the working heart. In the case of a heart attack, a blood clot develops and disrupts blood flow. If blood flow is not reestablished then a person can die. This event is referred to as a myocardial infarction, or heart attack.

RISK FACTORS FOR CARDIOVASCULAR DISEASE

To understand the concept of risk factors, it is important to understand what a risk factor is. Diseases such as cardiovascular disease are influenced by a variety of factors that can be divided into modifiable and non-modifiable categories. Non-modifiable risk factors are age, family history of heart disease, being a male, and race. Modifiable risk factors are those areas that can be affected by lifestyle modification: smoking, hypertension, dyslipidemia (cholesterol, LDL, HDL), type II diabetes mellitus, obesity, and a sedentary lifestyle. Table 19.1. Following is a brief description of CVD risk factors.

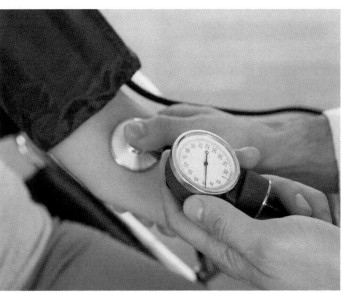

TABLE 19.1

Risk Factors for Cardiovascular Disease

Modifiable Risk Factors:
• Cigarette Smoking
• High Blood Pressure (Hypertension)
• High Blood Cholesterol
• Physical Inactivity
• Obesity and Overweight
• T2 Diabetes Mellitus
Non-Modifiable Risk Factors:
• Increasing Age
• Male Sex
• Race
• Heredity (Family History)

MESSAGE FROM A FORMER SMOKER

As a past smoker I tried many different strategies to quit. Once I finally quit, I wanted to avoid weight gain and didn't want to go back to being a smoker. I credit exercise with my success. Even though I smoked, I was a jogger. When I quit, I started jogging more. The extra exercise not only helped my health, but also made me not want to smoke. September 19, 1980, was my stop smoking day. I continue to be a non-smoker, and I continue to exercise. I credit exercise with my success. And I didn't gain any weight. If you want to stop, then look to exercise as a way to become a non-smoker. — Mike McCammon

MODIFIABLE CVD RISK FACTORS

CIGARETTE SMOKING

Cigarette smoking is considered a primary CVD risk factor and is related to heart disease risk in a dose-dependent manner. This means that the more you smoke the greater your risk of developing CVD. For each pack smoked per day the risk of coronary heart disease doubles. Sudden death from heart attacks is five times more common in smokers than in non-smokers. When cigarette smoking is combined with other risk factors, like high blood pressure and high blood cholesterol, the risk increases exponentially.

The best advice is to stop smoking. If you have tried to quit before and failed, do not be discouraged. On average, habitual smokers who eventually quit smoking quit five times before they stop smoking for good. For some individuals it may take more than five times, but it is worth the effort. Within two years of smoking cessation, CVD mortality risk declines markedly. Ten years after quitting, your risk is about the same as if you have never smoked. For most people smoking is incompatible with regular aerobic activity. If you do smoke, the beginning of a physical activity program may be an optimal time for you to stop smoking. Even though smoking is a

risk factor, smoking and being sedentary is a double risk whammy. If you're going to smoke, you need to exercise. While exercise doesn't take away smoking risk, it does provide protection for those that smoke.

Many people have been discouraged from quitting smoking due to a fear of gaining weight. However, weight gain is not as common as you might think. Also, individuals who increase their physical activity level can prevent or minimize weight gain associated with smoking cessation. Twenty to 30 minutes of daily exercise can reduce urges to smoke and eat. Exercise can be a key component for keeping your weight stable, and as an aid to keep you from starting to smoke again.

How exercise counteracts weight gain is interesting. While it is common knowledge that smoking blunts appetite, it also increases energy expenditure. Smoking results in an increase in metabolic rate. A pack-a-day smoker might expend an additional 200 Kcals/day. To counteract the smoking-related caloric expenditure, ex-smokers should start an exercise program. Exercise is a powerful tool in preventing weight gain. By exercising 20 to 30 minutes per day, it is possible to avoid smoking-cessation weight gain due to the calories expended through exercise.

Two other smoking-related issues should be noted: use of smokeless tobacco products and the effects of passive smoking. Use of smokeless tobacco products (chewing tobacco and snuff) has increased. However, many adverse health effects result from such use. Use of smokeless tobacco is associated with an increase in oral cancer and oral health problems, including halitosis (bad breath), gum recession, teeth abrasion, and periodontal bone loss. In addition, smokeless tobacco is associated with cardiovascular system, reproduction, and oral health problems, along with an overall decreased life expectancy. Passive smoking is the exposure to someone else's tobacco smoke, and this is also not without risk. Exposure to passive smoke increases the risk of lung cancer, heart disease, and respiratory diseases. In addition, children of smokers are likely to experience respiratory infections.

HIGH BLOOD PRESSURE

Blood pressure is the force exerted by the blood against the arterial wall. Systolic blood pressure represents the pressure in the arteries during contraction of the heart. Diastolic blood pressure is the pressure in the arteries during the relaxation or filling phase. Blood pressure is measured in millimeters of mercury (mmHg) and is expressed as systolic blood pressure over diastolic blood pressure (e.g., 120/80 mmHg).

A resting blood pressure value below 120/80 mmHg is considered normal and is typically associated with good health. Systolic blood pressure values between 120 and 139 mmHg, or diastolic blood pressure values between 80 and 89 mmHg are categorized as prehypertension. People with prehypertension are more likely to develop high blood pressure unless they take action to prevent it.

The term hypertension refers to high blood pressure. Hypertension is defined as chronically elevated systolic blood pressure of ≥140 mmHg and/or diastolic blood pressure of ≥90 mmHg. The term "chronically elevated" indicates that hypertension should not be diagnosed on the basis of one measurement. Diagnosis of hypertension is done by a physician after repeated measurements.

The prevalence rate of hypertension is higher in men than in women and higher among African Americans than among Caucasians. The prevalence also increases with age. Over 60% of the adult population 65+ years have hypertension.

Treatments available to reduce high blood pressure include: weight reduction, alcohol restriction, sodium restriction, regular aerobic exercise, and medication.

Weight Reduction. Epidemiologic studies clearly show that excess body fat and hypertension are highly related. A strong association exists between increases in body weight and subsequent development of high blood pressure. Hypertensive individuals who are overweight may reduce their blood pressure with weight loss. This weight loss is best accomplished by a combination of caloric restriction and regular exercise to burn calories. If you are overweight and hypertensive, you should try to lose at least 3% of your body weight. Losing more might have more of an affect, but research has shown that even modest weight loss will improve one's blood pressure.

Alcohol Restriction. Excessive alcohol intake can lead to hypertension. People with hypertension (as well as anyone else) who drink should do so in moderation (i.e., no more than 24 ounces of beer or 8 ounces of wine daily for men and no more than 12 ounces of beer or 4 ounces of wine daily for women).

Sodium Restriction. Some hypertensive patients (those who are sodium sensitive) can control their blood pressure through proper sodium restriction (less than 1 teaspoon of table salt per day). It is difficult to identify people with hypertension who are sodium sensitive; therefore, sodium restriction is probably appropriate for all people with high blood pressure. It is important to examine the sodium content of processed, canned, and frozen foods since much of the sodium intake comes from prepared foods. As college students, you also need to be aware of the amount of sodium found in fast foods. If you consistently eat fast food, you are getting much more sodium in your diet than is recommended. The recommended daily amount is 2500 mg/day, which is approximately equal to 1 teaspoon.

Regular Aerobic Exercise. Regular aerobic exercise is important for weight control and is effective for reducing blood pressure in individuals with pre-hypertension and hypertension.

Medication. Several types of pharmacologic agents are effective in the treatment of high blood pressure. Blood pressure is one disease that is relatively easy to control. Along with diet and exercise, some people might require medication.

KEY POINT
The reduction of high blood pressure by any means will reduce the risk of strokes and heart attacks and prolong lives.

DYSLIPIDEMIA

High levels of total cholesterol and LDL and/or low HDL levels are associated with an increased heart disease risk. The National Cholesterol Education Program (NCEP) guidelines for a desirable total cholesterol level is fewer than 200 milligrams per deciliter of blood (mg/dL). However, several other noted experts recommend even lower levels of < 180 mg/dL. In general, the lower the total cholesterol level the lower the risk. Data from the Framingham Study, an important epidemiologic research study, suggests that for every 1% reduction in total cholesterol, a 2% reduction in heart attack risk can be expected. The Framingham Study has provided several other important considerations. First, individuals with total cholesterol levels lower than 150 mg/dL were typically free of atherosclerosis. Secondly, approximately 15% of the heart attacks occurred in people with total cholesterol less than 200 mg/dL. For these individuals it is important to consider several critical components of cholesterol.

In addition to cholesterol level, the type of cholesterol is also important to consider. To circulate in the blood, cholesterol must be wrapped in a protein blanket. This combination is called a lipoprotein. The major culprit in the development of clogged arteries is low density lipoprotein (LDL). LDL tends to adhere to the walls of damaged arteries and high levels of LDL are associated with elevated cardiovascular disease risk. A more positive or protective component of cholesterol is high density lipoprotein (HDL). It is thought that HDL helps to remove plaque from the arterial walls and transport it to the liver where it is metabolized and eliminated. Thus, HDL provides a risk reduction function with higher levels associated with a lower risk of heart disease. HDL levels lower than 40 mg/dL are considered low and represent a risk factor for heart disease. An HDL level > 60 mg/dL is a high level and is protective against heart disease.

One key to heart disease risk seems to be the ratio of total cholesterol to HDL (total cholesterol/HDL). A lower ratio indicates a more favorable risk profile. This means that some people with moderately high total cholesterol values might have a low risk if their HDLs are high. Conversely, some individuals with apparently low total cholesterol levels may have an elevated risk if their HDLs are low. A desirable ratio would be less than 3.5 for women and less than 4.0 for men, since few heart attacks occur in people with this profile. The absolute risk of having a heart attack diminishes as the ratio gets lower. HDL levels are increased through regular aerobic exercise and weight reduction.

The NCEP Guidelines for classification of heart disease risk based on total cholesterol and LDL cholesterol levels are provided in Table 19.2.

TABLE 19.2

National Cholesterol Education Program – Classification of Coronary Heart Disease Risk from Total Cholesterol and LDL Cholesterol

Classification	Total Cholesterol
Desirable	< 200 mg/dL
Borderline high	200 – 239 mg/dL
High	≥ 240 mg/dL
Classification	**LDL Cholesterol**
Optimal	< 100 mg/dL
Near or above optimal	100 – 129 mg/dL
Borderline high	130 – 159 mg/dL
High	160 – 189 mg/dL
Very High	≥ 190 mg/dL

KEY POINT

Trans fat, saturated fat, and cholesterol in a diet increase total cholesterol and LDL and most Americans should strive to eat fewer of these fats and cholesterol. Visit www.americanheart.org for more information.

PHYSICAL INACTIVITY

Physical inactivity is an important predictor of cardiovascular disease. Regular physical activity and higher levels of cardiovascular fitness can help control many of the other risk factors. As noted earlier, individuals who expend a sufficient number of calories through physical activity and exercise and have an adequate level of aerobic fitness lower their risk of developing CVD. Regular aerobic exercise can also help control blood pressure, diabetes, and obesity; and can increase levels of HDL.

KEY POINT

Adults should accumulate at least 150 minutes (2 hours and 30 minutes) a week of moderate-intensity or 75 minutes (1 hour and 15 minutes) a week of vigorous-intensity aerobic activity, or an equivalent combination of moderate and vigorous aerobic activity.

Obesity and Overweight. Obesity is defined as an excessive accumulation of fat. It is associated with numerous adverse health conditions, including: hypertension, type II diabetes, coronary heart disease, dyslipidemia, osteoarthritis, psychological maladjustments, increased risk of some forms of cancer, and a shortened life expectancy. Overweight is defined by body mass index and was covered in greater detail in Module 7. For people who are overweight, even modest weight loss of 3% to 10% can help reduce hypertension and high blood cholesterol.

The prevention of obesity by balancing caloric expenditure and caloric intake represents the ideal situation. The treatment of obesity is challenging, with few programs or individuals able to document a high degree of long-term success (e.g., maintaining weight loss for 5 years or longer). The results of several research studies on both children and adults suggest that obesity is more associated with inactivity than with overeating (although both or either may be a cause of obesity for a given individual). Obese people may not eat more than non-obese people, but they are less active.

Physical inactivity can be either a cause or result of obesity. However, results of exercise training studies show substantial changes in body composition consequent to training programs that have a frequency of 3 to 4 days per week. Regular physical activity is a major factor in the prevention and treatment of obesity.

And even for those who cannot lose and maintain weight loss, physical activity and exercise are extremely important. From a health risk perspective, higher levels of cardiorespiratory fitness are more important than fatness. Obese individuals who have a high level of cardiorespiratory fitness are less likely to die from heart disease than normal weight, unfit individuals. What this means is that it is better (from a health perspective) to be fit than thin!

TYPE II DIABETES MELLITUS

Diabetes is a disease in which the body does not produce or respond properly to insulin. Insulin is a hormone needed for daily life processes; it allows the body to use glucose for energy. When insulin is deficient, blood glucose levels rise. People with diabetes have trouble controlling blood glucose levels.

Long-term elevation of blood glucose is associated with numerous health problems, among them: eye disease (retinopathy), kidney disease (nephropathy), nerve damage (peripheral neuropathy), impaired circulation, increased amputation risk, and cardiovascular disease (especially an increased risk of stroke, particularly in women).

Two types of diabetes mellitus exist. Approximately 90 - 95% of the 18 million people with diabetes in the United States have type II. The other 5 - 10% have type I. Type 1 diabetes is the result of the body losing its ability to make insulin. Type II diabetes is characterized by a reduction in insulin action leading to high glucose levels.

Obesity and physical inactivity are major risk factors for type II diabetes. Other risk factors include advancing age, being African American or Hispanic, and a family history of the disease. As individuals become obese, they become insulin resistant; that is, more insulin is required to normalize blood glucose levels. Over time insulin resistance can lead to diabetes.

Exercise recommendations for type II diabetics vary based on the individual. Longer duration, lower intensity exercise activities appear to be just as effective as higher intensity, longer duration exercise. A minimum of 150 minutes of physical activity per week is recommended. Increasing duration to 300 minutes per week appears to result in added benefit.

NON-MODIFIABLE CVD RISK FACTORS

INCREASING AGE

A greater incidence of cardiovascular disease is found among older individuals. This is probably due to many factors, among them are that people typically gain body fat and become less active with age.

It should be kept in mind, however, that cardiovascular disease is not a disease of the aged. The atherosclerotic process begins early in life. This has been known for many years. In the 1950s, autopsies were performed on American soldiers who were killed in Korea. The average age of these soldiers was only 22 years, yet 77% of the autopsies revealed evidence of atherosclerosis. Proper preventive measures must be followed by people of every age.

Male Sex. In middle age, men have a higher incidence of cardiovascular disease than women. However, cardiovascular disease rates are increasing for women.

Additionally, the incidence of cardiovascular disease increases greatly in women after menopause.

> **KEY POINT**
> Although men have a higher incidence of cardiovascular disease than women, the leading cause of death for women is heart disease.

HEREDITY

People with a family history of cardiovascular disease are at a greater risk of contracting that disease. This genetic predisposition is probably related to physical inactivity and other unhealthy lifestyle characteristics that tend to run in families. Since a family history of disease cannot be altered it is especially important for individuals who have this risk factor to limit as many other risk factors as possible.

> **KEY POINT**
> Because family history of heart disease cannot be controlled, it is even more important to keep other risk factors under control if your brother, father, or grandfather had a heart attack before age 55, or your sister, mother, or grandmother had a heart attack before age 65.

FITNESS MATTERS: SUCCESS STORIES

WHAT STUDENTS SAY ABOUT THIS CLASS . . . .

These lectures have made me realize how important EXSS 1000 and health in general is. This class has impacted my decision to change my major from nursing to exercise physiology and later on to physical therapy. — Virginia P.

RACE

Caucasians have lower heart disease risk than African Americans, American Indians, and Mexican Americans. This higher risk is partially due to higher rates of obesity and diabetes for some ethnic/racial groups.

MULTIPLE CARDIOVASCULAR DISEASE RISK FACTORS

The risk for developing cardiovascular disease increases if risk factors are present. Importantly, if more than one risk factor is present (e.g., a person smokes, has hypertension, and a high blood cholesterol level), then the risk of heart disease increases exponentially. This is another good reason to control as many risk factors as possible.

LEADING CAUSES OF DEATH

Diseases of the heart represent the leading cause of death in the United States. Cardiovascular diseases, such as heart disease and stroke, account for about 40% of all deaths. About one out of every four Americans has some form of cardiovascular disease. Cardiovascular disease affects women as well as men, and is debilitating for many people in the prime of their life.

Although the percentage of deaths from heart disease is high, it has changed dramatically since 1900. In 1900, when many jobs still required moderate to high levels of physical activity, heart disease accounted for less than 10% of deaths. From that time to the 1950s, as America became more modernized and necessary physical activity declined, a steady increase in the percentage of deaths from heart disease was seen. From the mid-1950s to the present time, we have actually witnessed a decrease in the percentage of deaths due to heart disease.

SUMMARY

Many diseases result from a lack of physical activity. Heart disease is the leading cause of death in the U.S.

- Controllable cardiovascular disease risk factors include cigarette smoking, high blood pressure, high blood cholesterol, physical inactivity, obesity, and type II diabetes.

- Uncontrollable cardiovascular disease risk factors include increasing age, male sex, race, and heredity.

MODULE TWENTY
FLEXIBILITY AND STRETCHING

OBJECTIVES

- Define flexibility.
- Understand the importance of flexibility for overall health and wellness.
- Describe ways to improve flexibility.
- Identify types of flexibility exercises appropriate for your fitness level.

INTRODUCTION

At the beginning of the semester you performed various fitness tests, including flexibility. In this module we will define flexibility, discuss its importance for overall health and wellness, and describe ways to improve your flexibility.

Flexibility is defined as the ability to move a joint and use muscles surrounding that joint through their full range of motion without pain. Flexibility involves the muscles, tendons, and ligaments of a specific joint and may vary greatly from joint to joint (i.e., you may have adequate levels of flexibility in the lower back and hamstring region, but not in the shoulder girdle). Maintaining or increasing your flexibility is important and flexibility training should be incorporated into all fitness routines. Routine flexibility training helps to reduce risk of injury and enhance performance in physical activities and exercise. In addition, flexibility is extremely important to many skill-related physical performances, such as an overhead serve in volleyball or a layup in basketball. Table 20.1 lists some benefits associated with a well-designed flexibility program.

Gender and age affect one's level of flexibility. Women tend to be more flexible than men, while younger individuals tend to be more flexible than older adults. In the case of decreased flexibility in older adults, research suggests that a decrease in physical activity is the primary source for the change. As we get older we tend to be less physically active and therefore lose the ability to move through a complete range of motion.

TYPES OF FLEXIBILITY TRAINING

The most frequently used technique for increasing flexibility is **static stretching**. During static stretching, the exerciser will slowly stretch the joint until he or she feels mild discomfort. The exerciser will hold the stretch for approximately 10 to 30 seconds, then repeat 2–4 times, with a goal of 60 seconds per muscle group. Performing static stretches after a workout when the muscles are warmest is recommended to obtain maximal benefits.

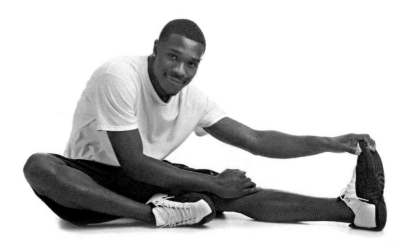

TABLE 20.1

Benefits of a Well-Designed Flexibility Program

- Increased physical performance
- Reduced muscle tension
- Maintenance of joint mobility
- Injury prevention
- Reduced stress

- Improved circulation
- Improved posture
- Enhanced muscle coordination
- Improved self-image
- Improved performance of ADLs

Another form of stretching is dynamic stretching, frequently used as part of a warm-up for any workout. Dynamic stretching is characterized by exercises designed to keep your body moving, focusing on large muscle groups moving through full range of motion (ROM). Examples of dynamic stretching include walking lunges, knee to chest lifts, body weight squats, and torso rotations. This type of stretching has gained much popularity over the last decade starting with sports teams and now is common in many types of fitness activities for all populations. According to numerous research studies, the benefits of dynamic stretching include:

- Increased core body temperature
- Increased blood supply to working muscles
- Increased ROM around joints

The purpose of dynamic stretching as part of an overall workout is to increase performance and decrease the risk of injury. Dynamic stretching involves movements that are specific to a sport or action. An example of dynamic stretching for a runner may be performing walking high knees or walking lunges. Both movements are specific to walking, jogging, or running and could be performed prior to engaging in such activities after a brief warm-up period (described below). Prior to strength training, slow controlled dynamic stretching provides movement rehearsal for complex exercises. While dynamic stretching does incorporate speed into the movements, this technique is different from **ballistic stretching** in that bouncing or jerking motions are avoided. Ballistic stretching is not recommended as an effective form of stretching, and should be avoided.

FLEXIBILITY PROGRAM DESIGN

When providing specific guidelines for designing a flexibility program, the literature is mixed at best. However, it is well accepted that a brief (5 to 10 minute bout of walking, slow jogging, cycling, or

FITNESS MATTERS: SUCCESS STORIES

WHAT STUDENTS SAY ABOUT THIS CLASS . . . .

I am a pretty active person but I didn't think that flexibility was too important. The flexibility lecture really taught me more about it and why it's important. — Dakota G.

I have learned new techniques for working different areas of the body. I have started doing stretches and exercises in my dorm with a towel. I'm starting to regain my flexibility. — Danielle D.

I injured my back two years ago and lost all my flexibility resulting from it. This lecture and yoga helped introduce me back into ways to regain flexibility. — Taylor C.

exercising on an elliptical machine) warm-up is beneficial before beginning any stretching program. This brief warm-up period helps to increase blood flow to the working muscles, thus improving the muscle's ability to stretch and reduces the possibility that injury will occur. You can compare this warm-up to starting your car on a cold winter morning. By doing so, you slowly raise the temperature of the engine (the muscles) and the oil (the blood) before you begin to drive (exercise).

We recommend static stretching as the primary mode of flexibility training. Current recommendations are to stretch a minimum of two to three days a week; however, like physical activity, daily is better. The intensity of your program should be that of mild discomfort or the point of tightness—stretching should not hurt! Finally, a well-designed flexibility program will incorporate all major muscle groups. If you are rehabbing an injury you may want to emphasize that specific muscle or joint, but still incorporate a full-body flexibility program. Table 20.2 describes a well-designed flexibility program using static stretching. Samples of common stretches are listed in the Flexibility and Stretching Appendix.

TABLE 20.2

Static Stretching Program Recommendations

- **Frequency:** 2–3 days a week, but daily is more effective
- **Intensity:** mild discomfort or point of tightness
- **Time:** 10–30 seconds with 2–4 repetitions, with a goal of accumulating 60 seconds per muscle group
- **Type:** all major muscle groups

SUMMARY

Maintaining or increasing flexibility is important for all fitness routines. Benefits of enhanced flexibility include improving physical performance, decreasing muscular tension, and preventing injuries.

MODULE TWENTY-ONE
ROADBLOCKS TO PHYSICAL ACTIVITY

OBJECTIVES

- Identify barriers to an active lifestyle.
- Explore a problem solving approach to overcome roadblocks.

INTRODUCTION

In earlier modules, you learned about self-monitoring, goal setting, and the ABCs of behavior change. Even by using those tools, becoming and staying physically active can be challenging. Each day we are faced with choices—some choices move us toward while others move us away from our healthy living goals. On the surface, becoming and staying physically active sounds easy—simply choose to make an active lifestyle a priority. However, the reality is that no matter how good our intentions, most of us experience roadblocks on the journey to an active lifestyle or in our quest to stay active. These challenges can be discouraging and take us off of our course for a while, but that's okay. That is part of the process. In this module we are going to examine barriers that stand in your way and how you can overcome them using a problem solving approach.

EXERCISE BARRIERS

Almost everyone can come up with reasons to NOT be physically active. **Exercise barriers** are all the factors that make exercise participation difficult and unattractive. Below are some common roadblocks or barriers to an active lifestyle. Do any of the reasons sound familiar?

I'd be more active if:

- I had more time
- The facilities were more conveniently located

- The facilities were less crowded
- I weren't so tired at the end of the day
- I didn't feel so self-conscious about how I looked when working out
- Physical activity were a higher priority in my life
- Exercising wasn't so fatiguing
- The weather was better for my favorite activities
- I was more skilled at fitness activities

If we brainstormed, we could probably come up with 100 different reasons that make physical activity participation difficult. However, you can find ways to get up, over, and around those barriers with a little creative thinking and planning. People who have a plan on how to overcome obstacles are more successful at staying active compared to those who

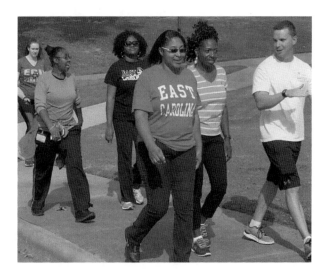

do not develop such a plan. For example, if time is an issue, choose a time during which you can make physical activity a priority or schedule it in your planner. If you are not naturally an early riser, don't schedule early morning workouts. Instead, exercise later in the day. If you can't motivate yourself to be active at home, don't bother investing in workout tapes. Instead, join a health club or exercise with a friend. Having a plan is a key to staying active even in the face of challenging circumstances. Below is a step-by-step plan that has helped others overcome exercise barriers.

Step 1: Identify the Barrier

This first step in overcoming barriers is to identify them. Take a moment and record roadblocks you either have experienced or anticipate experiencing on the path to achieving your goals and leading an active lifestyle.

ROADBLOCKS

Your Personal Barriers

1.

2.

3.

4.

5.

6.

7.

After you identified the barriers, circle the one or two most important barriers that are the most important roadblocks standing in your way of becoming or staying active and achieving your goals.

Step 2: Brainstorm Solutions

Brainstorm as many different strategies as you could use to overcome those barriers. What would it take for you to get past this barrier? In developing solutions, brainstorm several different strategies. You then have a better chance of finding a solution that works for you. To get you started in the brainstorming process, this chapter includes potential sample solutions to a couple of common barriers. However, you will probably be able to come up with better solutions that fit you and your lifestyle better than the ones listed. The key to brainstorming is to identify as many possible solutions as possible while withholding judgment on those solutions until later.

Recall the one or two most important barriers standing in your way that if overcome would help you achieve your goals. What are potential solutions to those barriers? Record as many ideas as possible.

_____

_____

_____

_____

_____

_____

Step 3: Evaluate Solutions

Look through the solutions you identified and decide which ones would help you the most. Evaluate how effective each solution would be in helping you overcome the barrier but also how feasible it is. Consider how likely, or unlikely, it will be that you actually carry out the solution. Getting up early in the morning to exercise might be an effective way to schedule exercise; it would not be very feasible if you are not a morning person. Once you have evaluated your potential solutions, circle the strategies that you will use this week.

Step 4: Put Your Plan into Action

Carry out the solution plan and then at the end of the week evaluate the results. Analyze how well your plan worked and revise if needed. If your plan worked well, give it a four-star rating. If it only deserves two stars, write down how it could become a four-star plan. If your plan didn't work at all, can you think of alternative strategies that you could use to get up, over, and around those roadblocks? A plan that

ROADBLOCKS AND POSSIBLE SOLUTIONS

Roadblocks	Possible Solutions
Example: Exercise takes too much time.	• I could try to gradually increase my daily activity by walking rather than taking the bus to my classes. • I will focus on the fact that a short walk re-energizes me and helps focus my attention so I use time more efficiently when active. • I could monitor my schedule and identify 30-minute time slots I could use for physical activity. • I could do 10 minutes of activity for a study break. • I could schedule time for activity in my day planner.
Example: Exercise is boring.	• I could ask a friend to work out with me. • I could try at least three different activities this week. • I could try recreational sports instead of exercise. • I could train for a 5K race.
Example: I feel self-conscious while exercising.	List your ideas on how a person could overcome this barrier.

does not work is not a failure—it often points to alternative solutions that will work.

_____

_____

_____

_____

_____

SUMMARY

In this module you learned about a problem solving approach to overcoming barriers.

One of the most important steps in overcoming barriers is to develop a healthy attitude about them. Recognize they are bound to happen. That is natural. But also recognize you have the ability to overcome them through effective problem solving. In many cases, it's not that physically active students experience fewer barriers than their less active counterparts. Rather, they experience similar barriers but have developed strategies to effectively deal with those barriers. We hope that this module provides you with the foundation for overcoming roadblocks that may stand in your way of an active lifestyle.

Want to learn more? Complete the Barriers to Being Active Quiz.

BARRIERS TO BEING ACTIVE QUIZ

What keeps you from being more active?

Directions: Listed below are reasons that people give to describe why they do not get as much physical activity as they think they should. Please read each statement and indicate how likely you are to say each of the following statements:

How likely are you to say?	Very likely	Somewhat likely	Somewhat unlikely	Very unlikely
1. My day is so busy now, I just don't think I can make the time to include physical activity in my regular schedule.	③	2	1	0
2. None of my family members or friends like to do anything active, so I don't have a chance to exercise.	3	2	1	⓪
3. I'm just too tired after work/school to get any exercise.	3	②	1	0
4. I've been thinking about getting more exercise, but I just can't seem to get started.	3	②	1	0
5. I'm injury prone.	3	2	1	⓪
6. I don't get enough exercise because I have never learned the skills for any sport.	3	2	1	⓪
7. I don't have access to jogging trails, swimming pools, bike paths, etc.	3	2	1	⓪
8. Physical activity takes too much time away from other commitments—time, work, family, etc.	3	②	1	0
9. I'm embarrassed about how I will look when I exercise with others.	3	2	①	0
10. I don't get enough sleep as it is. I just couldn't get up early or stay up late to get some exercise.	3	2	1	⓪
11. It's easier for me to find excuses not to exercise than to go out to do something.	3	2	①	0
12. I know of too many people who have hurt themselves by overdoing it with exercise.	3	2	1	⓪
13. I'm not coordinated enough to be successful at exercise.	3	2	1	⓪

BARRIERS TO BEING ACTIVE QUIZ (CONT.)

How likely are you to say?	Very likely	Somewhat likely	Somewhat unlikely	Very unlikely
14. It's just too expensive. You have to take a class or join a club or buy the right equipment.	3	2	(1)	0
15. My free times during the day are too short to include exercise.	3	2	1	(0)
16. My usual social activities with family or friends do not include physical activity.	3	2	(1)	0
17. I'm too tired during the week and I need the weekend to catch up on my rest.	3	(2)	1	0
18. I want to get more exercise, but I just can't seem to make myself stick to anything.	(3)	2	1	0
19. I'm afraid I might injure myself.	3	2	1	(0)
20. I'm not good enough at any physical activity to make it fun.	3	2	(1)	0
21. If exercise facilities were more convenient, then I would be more likely to exercise.	3	2	1	(0)

The Barriers to Being Active quiz is from *Promoting Physical Activity: A Guide for Community Action* (USDHHS, 1999).

BARRIERS TO BEING ACTIVE QUIZ: SCORING INSTRUCTIONS

Follow these instructions to score yourself:

Enter the circled number in the spaces provided, putting together the number for statement 1 on line 1, statement 2 on line 2, and so on.

Add the three scores on each line. Your barriers to physical activity fall into one or more of seven categories: lack of time, social influences, lack of energy, lack of willpower, fear of injury, lack of skill, and lack of resources. A score of 5 or above in any category shows that this is an important barrier for you to overcome.

$$\underset{1}{3} + \underset{8}{2} + \underset{15}{0} = 5 \qquad \text{Lack of time}$$

$$\underset{2}{0} + \underset{9}{1} + \underset{16}{1} = 2 \qquad \text{Social influence}$$

$$\underset{3}{2} + \underset{10}{0} + \underset{17}{2} = 4 \qquad \text{Lack of energy}$$

$$\underset{4}{2} + \underset{11}{1} + \underset{18}{3} = 6 \qquad \text{Lack of willpower}$$

$$\underset{5}{0} + \underset{12}{0} + \underset{19}{0} = 0 \qquad \text{Fear of injury}$$

$$\underset{6}{0} + \underset{13}{0} + \underset{20}{1} = 1 \qquad \text{Lack of skill}$$

$$\underset{7}{0} + \underset{14}{1} + \underset{21}{0} = 1 \qquad \text{Lack of resources}$$

SUGGESTIONS FOR OVERCOMING PHYSICAL ACTIVITY BARRIERS

Lack of time	Identify available time slots. Monitor your daily activities for one week. Identify at least three 30-minute time slots you could use for physical activity.
	Add physical activity to your daily routine. For example, walk or ride your bike to work or shopping, organize school activities around physical activity, walk the dog, exercise while you watch TV, park farther away from your destination, etc.
	Make time for physical activity. For example, walk, jog, or swim during your lunch hour, or take fitness breaks instead of coffee breaks.
	Select activities requiring minimal time, such as walking, jogging, or stairclimbing.
Social influence	Explain your interest in physical activity to friends and family. Ask them to support your efforts.
	Invite friends and family members to exercise with you. Plan social activities involving exercise.
	Develop new friendships with physically active people. Join a group, such as the YMCA or a hiking club.
Lack of energy	Schedule physical activity for times in the day or week when you feel energetic.
	Convince yourself that if you give it a chance, physical activity will increase your energy level; then, try it.
Lack of motivation	Plan ahead. Make physical activity a regular part of your daily or weekly schedule and write it on your calendar.
	Invite a friend to exercise with you on a regular basis and write it on both your calendars.
	Join an exercise group or class.
Fear of injury	Learn how to warm up and cool down to prevent injury.
	Learn how to exercise appropriately considering your age, fitness level, skill level, and health status.
	Choose activities involving minimum risk.

SUGGESTIONS FOR OVERCOMING PHYSICAL ACTIVITY BARRIERS (CONT.)

Lack of skill	Select activities requiring no new skills, such as walking, climbing stairs, or jogging. Find a friend who is willing to teach you some new skills. Take a class to develop new skills.
Lack of resources	Select activities that require minimal facilities or equipment, such as walking, jogging, jumping rope, or calisthenics. Identify inexpensive, convenient resources available in your community (community education programs, park and recreation programs, worksite programs, etc.).
Weather conditions	Develop a set of regular activities that are always available regardless of weather (indoor cycling, aerobic dance, indoor swimming, calisthenics, stair climbing, rope skipping, mall walking, dancing, gymnasium games, etc.). Look at outdoor activities that depend on weather conditions (cross-country skiing, outdoor swimming, outdoor tennis, etc.) as "bonuses"—extra activities possible when weather and circumstances permit.

FITNESS MATTERS: SUCCESS STORIES

WHAT STUDENTS SAY ABOUT THIS CLASS . . . .

They have allowed me to step out of my comfort zone and try new things! I use the exercise machines along with yoga. — Paige C.

I have begun faithfully working out thanks to this class and the above concepts. I use exercise machines, core and body weight training, and some yoga about 5 times a week. — Emilee B.

I now walk regularly on the trail way behind the dog park. — Meredith R.

MODULE TWENTY-TWO

UNDERSTANDING PHYSICAL ACTIVITY RECOMMENDATIONS

OBJECTIVES

- Understand how much physical activity is recommended based on guidelines provided by national organizations and why differing guidelines exist.
- Determine the type of physical activity and exercise program that is best for you based on your personal goals.

INTRODUCTION

How much physical activity and exercise do you need? If you read guidelines provided by various national organizations, you might be somewhat confused as the recommendations differ. The reason for these differences is because the optimal amount of activity depends on your goals. This module is designed to provide you with a better understanding of activity recommendations and a framework for making physical activity and exercise decisions.

For this module we focus on recommendations for adults without known cardiovascular or metabolic (diabetes, thyroid, etc.) disease. Even though many therapeutic benefits are associated with increasing activity levels, a small subset of the population with health issues should receive a thorough medical evaluation prior to initiating any form of physical activity.

Recommendations from the following organizations have been used to formulate physical activity/exercise suggestions:

- The American College of Sports Medicine (ACSM): http://acsm.org
- American Heart Association (AHA): www.heart.org
- Centers for Disease Control and Prevention (CDC): http://www.cdc.

gov/physicalactivity/everyone/guidelines/index.html
- National Institute of Health (NIH): http://www.nhlbi.nih.gov/health/health-topics/topics/phys/recommend.html
- International Association for the Study of Obesity (IASO): http://obesityepidemic.org/exercise recommendations.html
- Surgeon General (2010 report): http://www.cdc.gov/nccdphp/sgr/ataglan.htm
- World Health Organization (WHO): http://www.who.int/dietphysicalactivity/factsheet_adults/en

So how much activity do you need? The simple answer is that it depends on your goals and whether your focus is on improving health, fitness, and/or

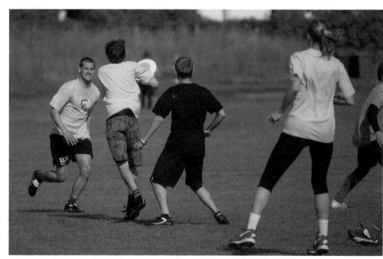

weight loss/maintenance. The different agencies recommendations have a common theme—more is better to a point! The key to exercise success is to determine your goals and then determine the best combination of time, duration, frequency, and intensity you can sustain now and in the future.

PHYSICAL ACTIVITY FOR HEALTH

If your goal is to improve or maintain health, several national organizations (e.g., American College of Sports Medicine, U.S. Department of Health and Human Services, Centers for Disease Control and Prevention, World Health Organization) recommend 150 minutes of moderate intensity activity per week or 5 days a week for 30 minutes. They also note comparable benefits can be accomplished through 75 minutes per week of vigorous activity, which can be accomplished by doing 25 minutes of vigorous aerobic activity at least 3 days per week. An equivalent mix of moderate- and vigorous-intensity aerobic activity can be used to meet recommendations for health benefits. Recall that moderate intensity activity is different than light activity in that your RPE should be between 3–5 during activity. A person doing vigorous-intensity activity will have an RPE of 6+. Health recommendations also highlight that short bouts (e.g., 10 minutes) that add up to 30 minutes have health benefits.

These recommendations are the minimum a person should strive to achieve to improve health. Additional health benefits can accrue with more activity, such as by increasing moderate-intensity activities to 5 hours (300 minutes) a week, or by increasing vigorous-intensity activity to 2 hours and 30 minutes per week. By increasing the duration and/or intensity of activities, greater health benefits will occur.

Meeting the minimum recommendations for health (150 minutes/week of moderate intensity activity) does not typically provide enough stimuli to promote substantial weight loss or fitness improvements for the average person.

EXERCISE FOR FITNESS

What if you want to develop cardiovascular fitness to improve performance or to achieve additional health benefits? Then you need to focus more on structured exercise to challenge (overload) the systems you want improved. If you want to improve your 5K run time, moderate intensity exercise will not adequately overload your cardiovascular system and promote

improved run times. Higher intensity, aerobic training that significantly challenges the body is associated with improvements in blood flow delivery and changes in how your body uses oxygen to produce ATP to do physical work.

In order to improve your fitness level, or in the case of improving your 5K run time, ACSM recommends the following using the FITTE principle:

- Frequency: 3 to 5 days/week
- Intensity: 60–85% of HRR or RPE 6+
- Time: 20–60 minutes per exercise bout
- Type: Recall the principle of specificity: If you want to run a blisteringly fast 5K you will need to run
- Enjoyment: activities that you like

In addition to aerobic exercise training, strength and flexibility training are also encouraged. You can find recommendations for these areas in Modules 12, 16, and 20.

> **KEY POINT**
> Start small and gradually increase the frequency, intensity, and duration to the level optimal to help achieve your personal goals. Keep in mind the dose-response relationship. If you increase the dose of the activity (i.e., intensity, duration, or frequency), then a greater fitness and health response will occur.

PHYSICAL ACTIVITY FOR WEIGHT CONTROL

As previously discussed, losing weight by focusing solely on increasing physical activity levels is unlikely. Successful weight loss and, more importantly, weight loss maintenance is dependent on changing eating patterns in addition to increasing physical activity levels. Several organizations (e.g., ACSM, IASO, NIH) highlight that 45 to 90 minutes of daily activity is needed lose weight or to prevent weight regain after losing weight.

FITNESS MATTERS: SUCCESS STORIES

WHAT STUDENTS SAY ABOUT THIS CLASS . . . .

These concepts taught me easy and affordable ways to exercise. This is very beneficial to a busy college student. — Rachel P.

They allowed me to not only talk about a subject, but to actually participate and recognize the benefits of particular programs. I'm still working on an exercise prescription program, but I plan to always stretch before activity. I may even consider doing yoga! — Jequetta T.

SRC group fitness, medicine balls and resistance bands, exercise machines, weight room, and body weight training were the most impactful because at first I was in a way scared to do these exercises and use the machines because I felt that I didn't know how to. These lectures and activities helped me know what to do. — Megan C.

Perhaps one way to evaluate the efficacy of physical activity on weight management is to review results obtained from the National Weight Control Registry (NWCR) (http://www.nwcr.ws). This registry is open to individuals who have maintained at least a 30-pound weight loss for at least one year. The NWCR provides information about registry participants in the fact section of their website. Not surprisingly, 94% report that they increased their physical activity and the most common form of activity chosen was walking. Furthermore, 90% reported that they average 60 minutes of daily activity.

Finding time and energy for 60-90 minutes of activity can be challenging. If that describes you, then consider accumulating 30 minutes of activity on 5 days per week. This will improve your health even if the numbers on the scale do not change. Health improvements can occur independent from weight loss. In addition, 30 minutes of physical activity can help with weight loss and maintenance when coupled with dietary change over a sustained period. If you don't have time for 60 to 90 minutes of daily activity, similar benefits can be achieved with 30-45 minutes of vigorous activity.

SUMMARY

So how much activity is recommended? It all depends on your goals and whether you are focused on improving health, increasing fitness for health and performance reasons, or on weight loss/maintenance. A core feature of most activity recommendations is that moderate intensity exercise provides health benefits independent of fitness improvement and weight loss in average fit individuals.

Weight loss/maintenance is enhanced by physical activity. Specifically, daily moderate intensity activity ranging from 45–90 minutes per day appears to have a positive effect on weight loss and maintenance, especially when combined with dietary changes.

PREVENTION AND CARE OF ATHLETIC INJURIES

OBJECTIVES

- Identify ways to prevent athletic injury
- Identify common athletic injuries
- Establish proper care of athletic injuries

INTRODUCTION

A common slogan used in health and fitness is, "no pain, no gain!" This slogan is a myth and can actually lead to an athletic injury. When participating in physical activity and exercise, your body should not be experiencing pain. Instead, you should be working at a level of intensity that is appropriate for your fitness level and at an intensity that will challenge your body without causing injury. Understanding the difference between pain and potential injury from intensity and fatigue is important when engaging in new exercises and activities and can be beneficial if you experience an athletic injury. Proper understanding of athletic injuries and the appropriate care that you should take will also be discussed in this module.

PREVENTION OF ATHLETIC INJURIES

Properly applying the FITT, progressive overload, and specificity principles is key to a successful fitness program in which your body will not only adapt and improve, but also avoid any injuries. As your fitness level increases your body will be able to sustain higher levels of exercise intensity, frequency, and time. Being in tune and mindful of how your body is responding to exercise will help you determine when you should progress in intensity and/or modify certain exercises. Choosing an appropriate exercise program or activity based on your level of fitness is the first step in preventing injuries.

If while participating in physical activity you experience pain or unusual discomfort in a certain part of your body that is affecting your performance, it is recommended that you evaluate this problem immediately. Remember, pain is not the same as fatigue or "feeling the burn" during an exercise. Pain is your body's way of telling you something isn't right. Your muscles, joints, or even bones are performing in a way that causes the body to respond with a clear signal that something is wrong and should be addressed immediately. "Feeling the burn" or properly applying the overload principle is different in that your body is still able to perform the movement or activity safely and with quality technique. While you will be fatigued and out of breath, you are not experiencing actual pain. See Table 1 for some common questions you can ask yourself to help determine if you are experiencing pain or properly fatiguing your body based on the principles you have learned in this class.

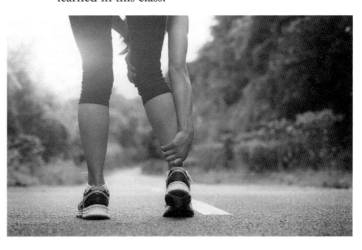

KEYPOINT

Listen to your body and understand the difference between pain and fatigue. Don't try to work through the pain and don't tell yourself, no pain no gain!

COMMON ATHLETIC INJURIES

Many injuries, both acute and chronic, can be a result of engaging in physical activity and exercise.

Acute injuries or pain refers to any sharp, specific pain that has a rapid onset and short duration. This type of injury is usually the result of a sudden incident that results in an injury to a specific part of the body. Common acute injuries include the following:

Fractures–cracks or breaks in bones; usually a cast is required to immobilize the bone.

Contusions–a bruise of the skin, fat, or muscle tissue resulting from a direct blow.

Sprains–stretching or tearing of a ligament, which connects bone to bone. Example: ankle sprain

Strains–stretching or tearing of a muscle, tendon, or fascial tissue. Example: hamstring strain.

Shoulder Dislocations–a fall or blow causes the top of your arm bone to pop out of the shoulder socket.

Dislocation–injury to a joint where the bones are forced out of normal position due to outside force (usually a fall or blow) and requires medical attention to return the bones to the proper position.

The opposite of acute pain or injury is chronic pain and injury. **Chronic injury** is a physical injury, illness, or disease that develops slowly over time and is persistent and long lasting, or constantly recurs over time. Chronic injuries are also referred to as overuse injuries. These injuries are usually a result of repetitive use, stress, and trauma or training errors. Common chronic injuries include the following:

TABLE 23.1

Questions to Determine if You Are Experiencing a Potential Injury vs. Muscular Fatigue

- Is this a new feeling that I haven't experienced before?

- Do I only experience it while performing a certain activity or exercise?

- Is this feeling preventing me from completing normal daily activities such as walking, taking stairs, etc.?

- Have I felt this feeling before? If so, is the feeling worse than when I previously felt it?

- Have I had this feeling in the past and does it keep recurring?

- Does the feeling continue long after the exercise or activity has stopped?

If you answered yes to several of these questions it is suggested that you seek medical attention. Injuries should be evaluated by a medical professional, such as an athletic trainer, physician, and/or physical therapist.

Tendinitis–inflammation of a tendon, which connects muscle to bone. Example: patella tendinitis.

Stress Fracture–caused by repetitive stress applied to a bone resulting in tiny cracks. Commonly affects weight-bearing bones of the lower extremity.

Shin Splints–pain along the tibia (also known as shinbone). This injury is common in runners and dancers, frequently due to increasing intensity or change in training that overloads the muscles and tendons.

Plantar Fasciitis–common with individuals who are on their feet a lot, either through physical activity and/or their occupation. The fascial tissue supporting the arch of the foot becomes inflamed and sore.

TREATMENT AND CARE OF INJURIES

When experiencing an acute injury, immediate medical attention is usually required either through first aid treatment and/or from a physician. After medical treatment has been issued, treating an acute injury is a simple as applying RICE. **RICE** is an acronym for Rest, Ice, Compression, and Elevations and is used to treat injuries such as sprains and fractures.

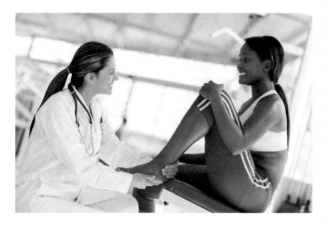

Rest, giving your body time to heal, is crucial to allow recovery from an acute injury. Avoiding exercises and activities that will further stress the injury you experienced is recommended.

Ice can provide short-term pain relief to an injured or inflamed area. It will help decrease swelling by decreasing the amount of blood flow to the injured area of the body. Ice should not be applied directly to the skin; instead, a towel or paper towel should be placed over the injured area before applying ice for 15–20 minutes every 2–3 hours.

Compression helps to prevent swelling in the injured area. Wrapping the area with a bandage is a way to apply consistent compression and provide stabilization to a weakened joint. For example using an ACE bandage with an ankle sprain will compress the injured area and help limit swelling.

Elevation helps control blood flow to the area and thus reduce swelling. Elevating the injured area above heart level is most effective.

The RICE method can also be applied when caring for chronic injuries. Further action and attention may be necessary in the form of surgeries, physical therapy, and rehabilitation of the injured area. If you suspect you are suffering from chronic pain or injury, talk with your instructor and seek advanced medical attention.

SUMMARY

Finding activities that you enjoy is important when adopting a healthy lifestyle that you can maintain throughout the college years and beyond. Engaging in these activities and exercises safely is the key to avoiding an athletic injury. See Table 2 for safety tips to help avoid and prevent an athletic injury. Table 3 outlines common signs for both acute and chronic athletic injuries. If an athletic injury of any kind is suspected be sure to take the appropriate steps for care and recovery, talk with your instructor or seek advanced medical attention.

TABLE 23.2

Safety Tips to Help Prevent Injuries

- Don't be a "weekend warrior." Don't try to do a weeks' worth of activity in a day or two.

- Know your body's limits.

- Gradually build up your exercise level.

- Strive for a total body workout of cardiovascular, strength training, and flexibility exercises.

- Do warm-up exercises before you play any sport or physical activity.

- Cool down after hard sports or workouts.

- Wear shoes that fit properly, are stable, and absorb shock.

- When jumping, always land with your knees bent.

TABLE 23.3

Common Signs of Acute and Chronic Injuries

Signs of an acute injury include:

- Sudden, severe pain.
- Swelling.
- Not being able to place weight on a leg, knee, ankle, or foot.
- An arm, elbow, wrist, hand, or finger that is very tender.
- Not being able to move a joint normally.
- Extreme leg or arm weakness.
- A bone or joint that is visibly out of place.

Signs of a chronic injury include:

- Pain when you play.
- Pain when you exercise.
- A dull ache when you rest.
- Swelling.

MODULE TWENTY-FOUR
KEEPING IT GOING AFTER THE SEMESTER IS OVER

OBJECTIVES

- Review some of the tools you have learned throughout the semester.
- Develop a plan for staying active now that the semester is coming to a close.

INTRODUCTION

We hope you enjoyed Kinesiology 1000 and learned skills that can help you lead a physically active lifestyle. No single approach to lifestyle change works for everyone. Each person is unique. Our goals this semester were to help you become more aware of your fitness levels, to provide you knowledge on how to structure an exercise program personalized to meet your objectives, and to provide tools to help you on the journey to an active lifestyle.

An important point is to recognize that no matter how dedicated you are, you will probably hit rough patches along the way that make it difficult to stick with your activity plan. Everyone does. For some it's the holiday season, for others it's a crazy schedule at school. Other people may be thrown off schedule by an illness or an injury. Even a change of schedule like the end of the semester can disrupt your exercise routine. Whatever the cause, there are going to be times when it's challenging to maintain your activity plan.

Having a lapse (i.e., missing a few days of exercise) at some point is unavoidable and natural. But we want to arm you with some strategies that will keep those temporary lapses from turning into a complete relapse that result in your discontinuing exercise.

The first strategy is to recognize that lapses are natural. Perhaps you do miss a few days. That does not mean you've failed, rather it means you had a lapse. One of the biggest mistakes people make when they miss a few days of activity is to fall into the all-or-nothing trap. They think "I'm either on my program or off my program. I just missed a few days so that means I'm off my program." Or they may think "I'm just not cut out to be active and doomed to be a couch potato. I don't have the willpower to stick to my goals so why try." Don't believe it. A lapse does not mean you are destined to be a couch potato or that you failed. Rather, it means you have missed a few days. Not all is lost. You just need to get started back on track.

How do you get back on track? The second strategy to preventing a relapse is to use the tools you have learned this semester.

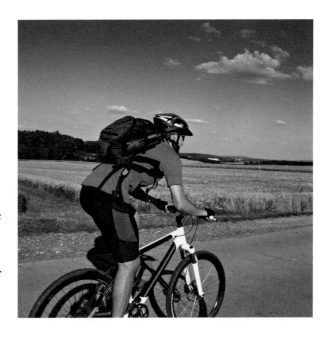

FITNESS MATTERS: SUCCESS STORIES

WHAT STUDENTS SAY ABOUT THIS CLASS . . . .

These concepts have impacted me throughout the course because I have learned a lot about exercises that I wouldn't have tried outside the class. I now am less hesitant to try something new in my exercise routine. Before this class I only did cardio exercises, now I incorporate resistance bands into my routine. I went and bought them because of this class. — Jessica M.

The concepts I circled are all activities that I could do to stay physically active without having to go to the gym. When I get older, I may not have the luxury of going to the gym, but I can still find a way to stay active. — Alicia G.

Group fitness day made me realize that exercising can be fun and enjoyable. — Tiffany M.

- Remember how being active benefits you personally. An active lifestyle will improve and maintain your health and quality of life. It can help you feel better. It can also lower stress and improve mood and energy.

- Find creative ways to incorporate enjoyable activity into your lifestyle.

- Continue to self-monitor your activity levels (and how much time you spend in sedentary behavior) or if you are getting off track, start self-monitoring again.

- Develop SMART goals.

- Apply problem solving skills to overcome exercise barriers.

- Use the ABCs of behavior change. For example, use your self-talk to motivate you. Increase cues (e.g., put your running shoes by your door) and decrease antecedents prompting inactivity.

- Include your favorite dissociation techniques.

- Develop an exercise contract for yourself.

The third strategy is to anticipate situations that may derail your efforts to stay active and plan for them. Sometimes a lapse strikes from nowhere. Maybe you've had an injury or have been under the weather. Or perhaps some other unforeseen event occurred. However, many lapses are predictable and can be anticipated. As long as you know which situations may cause problems and make it difficult to stick with your program, you can avoid being sidetracked by planning for them.

PLANNING FOR CHALLENGES

Many challenging situations or obstacles exist. Can you anticipate any situations that may disrupt your exercise routine? Describe those situations below.

High-Risk Situations

Example: The semester is coming to an end and you will not be enrolled in KINE 1000.

1. _____
   _____
   _____

2. _____
   _____
   _____

Now, develop a plan of action for dealing with that challenging situation by developing a plan that is specific and realistic for you. What plan can you make now to stay on track? Students who anticipate and plan are better able to deal with challenging situations compared to those who wait until after the fact to get back on track.

Strategies for Dealing with Challenging Situations

Example: I will schedule when I will exercise in my planner after break so missing a few days doesn't cause me to stop my exercise program completely.

1. _____
   _____
   _____

2. _____
   _____
   _____

Imagine you do have a lapse and do take a temporary "break." What strategies will help you get started again? Write down your ideas.

Jump Start Ideas _____

_____

_____

_____

_____

SUMMARY

We've said it before, but it's worth repeating—we hope you are physically active for the long haul. The path to an active lifestyle seems simple and straightforward: Just get off the couch and move. As simple as that may sound, sticking with an exercise program is difficult for many. One of the most important things to remember is that motivation is easier if you are doing something you enjoy, so do not overlook the importance of finding activities you enjoy. Also, remember, your goal is not to get fit overnight; you want to adopt a lifelong physically active lifestyle. Use self-monitoring, goal planning, problem solving to overcome barriers, and the ABCs of behavior change to help make that process easier. As you continue your journey to an active lifestyle, find motivation from your successes and recognize that experiencing difficulties and occasional setbacks is part of the process. Not only can you use the skills you have learned to increase your activity level, these skills can be applied to other areas in your life as well, such as improving your dietary habits, smoking cessation, and time management. The success of these behavior change strategies depends on you. The more you use and apply them, the more you will benefit from them. The road to a healthy, active lifestyle begins with a single step. Are you ready?

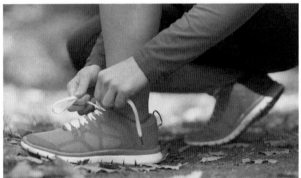

INITIAL FITNESS TESTING LAB EXPERIENCE: WOMEN

Name_____ Class_____ Hour _____

Gender _____ Age _____ Height_____ Weight_____

Test	Healthy Fitness Zone	Your Score	Achieved HFZ? (Yes/No)
Aerobic Fitness			
PACER (# of laps completed)	≥ 38	_____	_____
VO$_2$ max (mL·kg^{-1}·min^{-1})	≥ 38.6	_____	_____
Body Composition			
Percent Fat (%)	16.5 – 31.3%	_____	_____
Abdominal Strength and Endurance			
Curl-ups (# completed)	≥ 18	_____	_____
Upper Body Strength and Endurance			
Push-ups (# completed)	≥ 7	_____	_____
Flexibility			
Sit-and-reach (inches)			
Right leg	12	_____	_____
Left leg	12	_____	_____
Shoulder Stretch			
Right side	Touch finger together behind back		
Left side		_____	_____

APPENDIX ONE

FITNESS TESTING LAB EXPERIENCE: WOMEN

Name_____ Class_____ Hour _____

Gender _____   Age _____   Height_____   Weight_____

Test	Healthy Fitness Zone	Your Score	Achieved HFZ? (Yes/No)
Aerobic Fitness			
PACER (# of laps completed)	≥ 38	_____	_____
VO$_2$ max (mL·kg^{-1}·min^{-1})	≥ 38.6	_____	_____
Body Composition			
Percent Fat (%)	16.5 – 31.3%	_____	_____
Abdominal Strength and Endurance			
Curl-ups (# completed)	≥ 18	_____	_____
Upper Body Strength and Endurance			
Push-ups (# completed)	≥ 7	_____	_____
Flexibility			
Sit-and-reach (inches)			
Right leg	12	_____	_____
Left leg	12	_____	_____
Shoulder Stretch			
Right side	Touch finger together behind back		
Left side		_____	_____

INITIAL FITNESS TESTING LAB EXPERIENCE: MEN

Name_____ Class_____ Hour _____

Gender _____ Age _____ Height_____ Weight_____

Test	Healthy Fitness Zone	Your Score	Achieved HFZ? (Yes/No)
Aerobic Fitness			
PACER (# of laps completed)	≥ 44	_____	_____
VO_2 max ($mL \cdot kg^{-1} \cdot min^{-1}$)	≥ 44.3	_____	_____
Body Composition			
Percent Fat (%)	$7 - 22\%$	_____	_____
Abdominal Strength and Endurance			
Curl-ups (# completed)	≥ 24	_____	_____
Upper Body Strength and Endurance			
Push-ups (# completed)	≥ 18	_____	_____
Flexibility			
Sit-and-reach (inches)			
Right leg	8	_____	_____
Left leg	8	_____	_____
Shoulder Stretch			
Right side	Touch finger together behind back		
Left side		_____	_____

APPENDIX TWO

FITNESS TESTING LAB EXPERIENCE: MEN

Name_____ Class_____ Hour _____

Gender _____ Age _____ Height_____ Weight_____

Test	Healthy Fitness Zone	Your Score	Achieved HFZ? (Yes/No)
Aerobic Fitness			
PACER (# of laps completed)	≥ 44	_____	_____
VO$_2$ max (mL·kg^{-1}·min^{-1})	≥ 44.3	_____	_____
Body Composition			
Percent Fat (%)	7 – 22%	_____	_____
Abdominal Strength and Endurance			
Curl-ups (# completed)	≥ 24	_____	_____
Upper Body Strength and Endurance			
Push-ups (# completed)	≥ 18	_____	_____
Flexibility			
Sit-and-reach (inches)			
Right leg	8	_____	_____
Left leg	8	_____	_____
Shoulder Stretch			
Right side	Touch finger together behind back	_____	_____
Left side			

ALTERNATIVE PHYSICAL FITNESS ASSESSMENTS

MILE RUN

The objective of this test is to cover a 1-mile course as quickly as possible. Results from the Mile Run test can then be compared to the standards in Table 6.1 to determine whether your aerobic fitness is in the Healthy Fitness Zone or whether you need improvement in this area.

The Mile Run test is a maximal test, and thus should only be attempted by young (< 45 years old for men and < 55 years old for women) and healthy individuals. The test should not be used with individuals who have known heart disease or symptoms of heart disease, such as chest discomfort that results from physical exertion.

The ability to pace yourself is an essential skill for this test. Best results are usually obtained when you maintain a steady pace throughout the test, as opposed to running too fast at the beginning and then needing to slow dramatically due to fatigue. Knowledge of pace is usually accomplished with several weeks of practice before testing takes place.

The only items needed to conduct the test are a measured 1-mile course (such as 4 laps around a school track) and a stopwatch.

PROCEDURES FOR THE MILE RUN

1. Warm-up appropriately. Begin with low intensity activity, such as walking or slow jogging, designed to increase blood flow to the muscles that you will be using. Then perform some stretching exercises.

2. Have a partner ready to count your laps (if you are running around a track).

3. Try to cover 1 mile in the fastest possible time. You may walk or jog or use a combination thereof. You should be reasonably exhausted at the end of the test. The faster the distance is covered the higher the estimated aerobic fitness.

4. Upon completion of the test, cool down for as long as necessary with slow jogging and/or walking (usually for 4 to 7 minutes). Then perform some stretching exercises. Do not sit or lie down immediately after the test. Sitting immediately after heavy exertion can allow the blood to pool in the legs and make you lightheaded.

5. Record your time to complete the mile. Estimate your VO_{2max} with the following formula:

$$VO_{2max}\ (mL \cdot kg^{-1} \cdot min^{-1}) = 108.94 - (8.41 \times time) + (0.34 \times time^2) + (0.21 \times age \times gender) - (0.84 \times BMI)$$

where time is mile run time in minutes, age is in years, gender is coded as 1 for male and 0 for female, and BMI is body mass index.

6. Indicate whether your score is in or above the Healthy Fitness Zone for VO_{2max} in Table 6.1 or whether your score indicates the need for improvement.

PROCEDURES TO ESTIMATE PERCENT FAT FROM SKINFOLDS

Have a trained tester measure skinfolds at the following sites:

Men	Women
Chest _____	Triceps _____
Abdomen _____	Suprailium _____
Thigh _____	Thigh _____
Sum _____	Sum _____

Sum the three skinfolds.

Refer to the tables on the following pages for your gender to estimate your percent fat from the sum of skinfolds, sex, and age.

Compare your percent fat to the standards provided in Table 7.2.

Estimates of Percent Fat for Women; Sum of Triceps, Suprailium, and Thigh Skinfolds

Sum of Skinfolds (mm)	Age in Years							
	20	25	30	35	40	45	50	55
22	9.8	10.1	10.4	10.7	11.0	11.3	11.6	11.9
25	11.0	11.3	11.6	11.9	12.2	12.5	12.8	13.1
28	12.1	12.4	12.7	13.0	13.3	13.6	13.9	14.2
31	13.2	13.5	13.8	14.1	14.4	14.7	15.0	15.3
34	14.3	14.6	14.9	15.2	15.5	15.8	16.1	16.4
37	15.4	15.7	16.0	16.3	16.6	16.9	17.2	17.5
40	16.5	16.8	17.1	17.4	17.7	18.0	18.3	18.6
43	17.5	17.8	18.1	18.4	18.8	19.1	19.4	19.7
46	18.6	18.9	19.2	19.5	19.8	20.1	20.4	20.7
49	19.6	19.9	20.2	20.5	20.8	21.2	21.5	21.8
52	20.6	20.9	21.2	21.6	21.9	22.2	22.5	22.8
55	21.6	21.9	22.3	22.6	22.9	23.2	23.5	23.8
58	22.6	22.9	23.2	23.6	23.9	24.2	24.5	24.8
61	23.6	23.9	24.2	24.5	24.9	25.2	25.5	25.8
64	24.6	24.9	25.2	25.5	25.8	26.1	26.5	26.8
67	25.5	25.8	26.1	26.5	26.8	27.1	27.4	27.7
70	26.4	26.7	27.1	27.4	27.7	28.0	28.4	28.7
73	27.3	27.7	28.0	28.3	28.6	29.0	29.3	29.6
76	28.2	28.6	28.9	29.2	29.5	29.9	30.2	30.5
79	29.1	29.5	29.8	30.1	30.4	30.7	31.1	31.4
82	30.0	30.3	30.6	31.0	31.3	31.6	31.9	32.3
85	30.8	31.2	31.5	31.8	32.2	32.5	32.8	33.1
88	31.7	32.0	32.3	32.7	33.0	33.3	33.6	34.0
91	32.5	32.8	33.2	33.5	33.8	34.1	34.5	34.8
94	33.3	33.6	34.0	34.3	34.6	35.0	35.3	35.6
97	34.1	34.4	34.7	35.1	35.4	35.7	36.1	36.4
100	34.9	35.2	35.5	35.9	36.2	36.5	36.8	37.2
103	35.6	35.9	36.3	36.6	36.9	37.3	37.6	37.9
106	36.3	36.7	37.0	37.3	37.7	38.0	38.3	38.7
109	37.1	37.4	37.7	38.1	38.4	38.7	39.1	39.4
112	37.8	38.1	38.4	38.8	39.1	39.4	39.8	40.1
115	38.4	38.8	39.1	39.4	39.8	40.1	40.5	40.8

Estimates of Percent Fat for Men; Sum of Chest, Abdomen, and Thigh Skinfolds

Sum of Skinfolds (mm)	Age in Years							
	20	**25**	**30**	**35**	**40**	**45**	**50**	**55**
16	3.5	4.1	4.6	5.2	5.7	6.2	6.8	7.3
19	4.5	5.0	5.6	6.1	6.7	7.2	7.7	8.3
22	5.5	6.0	6.5	7.1	7.6	8.2	8.7	9.3
25	6.4	6.9	7.5	8.0	8.6	9.1	9.7	10.2
28	7.3	7.9	8.4	9.0	9.5	10.1	10.6	11.2
31	8.3	8.8	9.4	9.9	10.5	11.0	11.6	12.1
34	9.2	9.7	10.3	10.8	11.4	12.0	12.5	13.1
37	10.1	10.7	11.2	11.8	12.3	12.9	13.4	14.0
40	11.0	11.6	12.1	12.7	13.2	13.8	14.4	14.9
43	11.9	12.5	13.0	13.6	14.1	14.7	15.3	15.8
46	12.8	13.4	13.9	14.5	15.0	15.6	16.2	16.7
49	13.7	14.2	14.8	15.4	15.9	16.5	17.1	17.6
52	14.5	15.1	15.7	16.2	16.8	17.4	17.9	18.5
55	15.4	16.0	16.5	17.1	17.7	18.2	18.8	19.4
58	16.2	16.8	17.4	18.0	18.5	19.1	19.7	20.2
61	17.1	17.7	18.2	18.8	19.4	19.9	20.5	21.1
64	17.9	18.5	19.1	19.6	20.2	20.8	21.4	21.9
67	18.7	19.3	19.9	20.5	21.0	21.6	22.2	22.8
70	19.5	20.1	20.7	21.3	21.9	22.4	23.0	23.6
73	20.3	20.9	21.5	22.1	22.7	23.2	23.8	24.4
76	21.1	21.7	22.3	22.9	23.5	24.0	24.6	25.2
79	21.9	22.5	23.1	23.7	24.2	24.8	25.4	26.0
82	22.7	23.3	23.9	24.4	25.0	25.6	26.2	26.8
85	23.4	24.0	24.6	25.2	25.8	26.4	27.0	27.6
88	24.2	24.8	25.4	26.0	26.5	27.1	27.7	28.3
91	24.9	25.5	26.1	26.7	27.3	27.9	28.5	29.1
94	25.7	26.2	26.8	27.4	28.0	28.6	29.2	29.8
97	26.4	27.0	27.6	28.2	28.7	29.3	29.9	30.5
100	27.1	27.7	28.3	28.9	29.5	30.1	30.7	31.3
103	27.8	28.4	29.0	29.6	30.2	30.8	31.4	32.0
106	28.5	29.1	29.6	30.2	30.8	31.4	32.1	32.7
109	29.1	29.7	30.3	30.9	31.5	32.1	32.7	33.3
112	29.8	30.4	31.0	31.6	32.2	32.8	33.4	34.0
115	30.4	31.0	31.6	32.2	32.8	33.5	34.1	34.7

APPENDIX FOUR

MUSCULAR STRENGTH

ASSESSMENT OF MUSCULAR STRENGTH: PERFORMING A 1-REPETITION MAXIMUM (1-RM)

After a brief warm-up utilizing lighter weights (usually starting with 50% of the estimated 1-RM and increasing the load based on the difficulty of the previous load), participants are instructed to lift as much weight as possible during a single repetition keeping the proper form and range of motion (ROM). The achievement of the 1-RM test should be completed within one to four sets because fatigue may begin to affect performance. If more than four sets are required, the test should be stopped and resumed another day after adequate rest (usually one week later). **Note: Before beginning any type of maximal resistance training exercise, always make sure that you have a qualified spotter to guarantee that proper form and safety are not compromised while executing the exercise.**

ASSESSMENT OF MUSCULAR STRENGTH: PERFORMING AN 8- TO 15-REPETITION MAXIMUM (RM)

An indirect method for determining an individual's 1-RM can be accomplished by performing an 8- to 15-RM test using a submaximal load. Although, you are using a submaximal load, an 8- to 15-RM test requires that a maximal number of repetitions be performed, thus making this technique a maximal test. Directions for assessing an 8- to 15-RM are similar to a 1-RM, but individuals should use a load that will cause fatigue within 8 to 15 repetitions (roughly 65 to 80% less than the estimated 1-RM). If an individual can perform more than 15 repetitions, the load should be increased and repeated after a full recovery. **Note: Before beginning any type of maximal resistance training exercise, always make sure that you have a qualified spotter to guarantee that proper form and safety are not compromised while executing the exercise.**

Use the table below to estimate your 1-RM from an 8- to 15-RM assessment. The table below depicts the percentage of 1-RM and 8- to 15-RM relationship. Simply take the submaximal load lifted during the assessment and divide it by the appropriate percentage (in a decimal form) depending on the number of repetitions performed. For example, let us say that you wanted to estimate lower body maximal strength with a standard leg press using a submaximal load of 100 pounds. After a brief warm-up with a lighter load, you performed 12 repetitions with 100 pounds on the leg press. Using the table you know that 12 repetitions is associated with roughly 67%, or 0.67, of your 1-RM. If you divide 100 pounds by 0.67, your estimated 1-RM would be 149.25 pounds or 149 pounds. This estimate of maximal strength will be helpful when designing your own resistance training routine.

Relationship between Repetitions Performed and % of 1 RM

% 1-RM	Estimated number of repetitions
100	1
80	8
77	9
75	10
70	11
67	12
65	15

The bench press and machine chest press are common lifts for assessing upper-body muscular strength utilizing either a 1-RM or an 8- to 15-RM test. The squat and machine leg press are common lifts for assessing lower-body muscular strength.

Examples of common exercises used to strength and tone different muscles of the body are listed on the following pages. Please read the description of each exercise before beginning your own resistance training program. Also refer to figures of the anterior muscles and posterior muscles when determining which muscles or groups of muscles are used with each exercise.

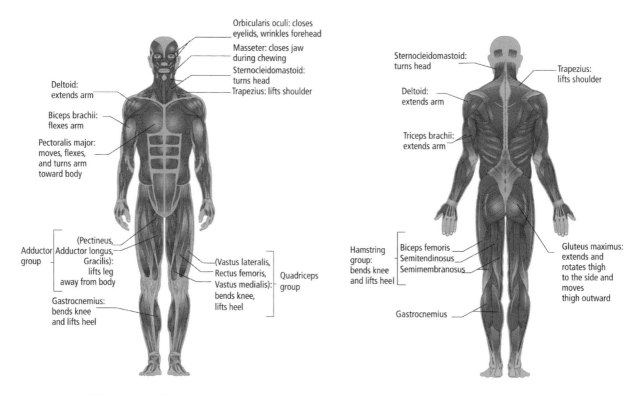

Anterior and Posterior Muscles

LOWER-BODY EXERCISES

Exercise	Number of Joints and Muscle Groups Involved	Description
Leg Press	**Multi-joint:** Hip and Knee **Primary:** Quadriceps **Secondary:** Gluteus Maximus and Hamstrings	Position your feet on the foot plate slightly wider than shoulder width. Your toes may point straight ahead or slightly outward. After you are in position, push the foot plate upward and release safety bars with both handles (top figures). In a controlled motion, lower the weight by bending the knees until roughly 90 degrees of flexion, then extend your knees and return to the initial position. At the top you want to avoid locking your knees to prevent hyperextension. Repeat through completion of set. After completing set, turn handles in to engage safety bars (top right figure) and lower weight.

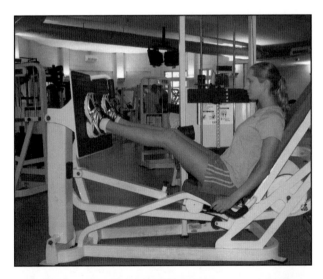

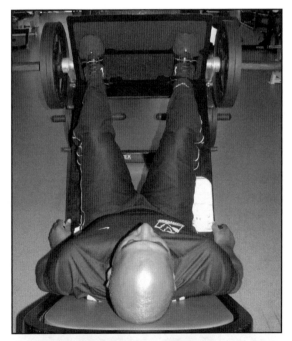

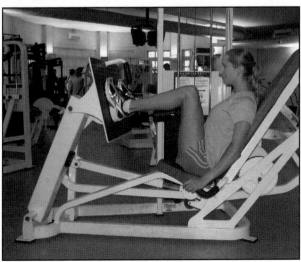

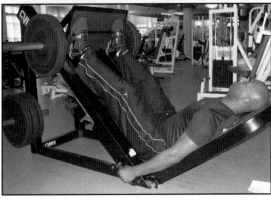

LOWER-BODY EXERCISES

Exercise	Number of Joints and Muscle Groups Involved	Description
Squat	**Multi-joint:** Hip and Knee **Primary:** Quadriceps **Secondary:** Gluteus Maximus and Hamstrings	Position your feet on the floor slightly wider than shoulder width. Your toes should be pointed slightly outward. After your feet are in position, grasp the bar with your hands and slide your head and shoulders under the bar. Place the bar along your trapezius muscle by pulling your shoulder blades back. Keeping your chest out and abdominal muscles tight, slowly stand upright raising the bar from the rack. Take two to three small steps back and assume the same foot position described earlier. Slowly allow your knees and hips to flex keeping your heels in contact with the floor at all times. During this downward movement, do not allow your knees to go beyond your toes. Also, it is important not to flex the spine (round the back). Continue flexing the hips and spine until your quadriceps are parallel to the floor. At this point, begin to extend the hips and thighs by applying force through your heels (not toes). At the top of the movement you want to avoid full extension (avoid locking your knees). Repeat until desired repetitions are complete and rack the weight.

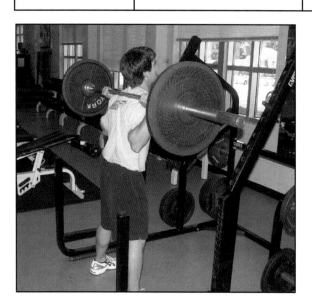

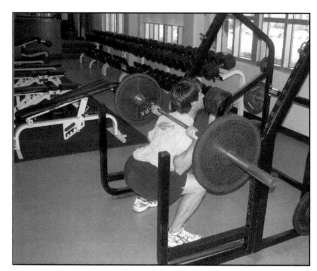

LOWER-BODY EXERCISES

Exercise	Number of Joints and Muscle Groups Involved	Description
Lunges	**Multi-joint:** Hip and Knee **Primary:** Quadriceps **Secondary:** Gluteus Maximus and Hamstrings	With feet together (stance), take an exaggerated step forward, keeping your back straight and chest out. Slowly lower your body until your front knee is flexed 90 degrees and your thigh is parallel to the floor. Your back leg will bend towards the floor, but avoid banging your knee on the ground. With your front heel on the ground, drive your weight upwards by pressing through your heel and bring back leg forward to stance. Repeat with other leg until you have completed the desired number of repetitions.

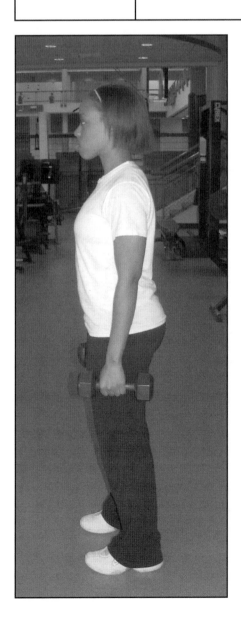
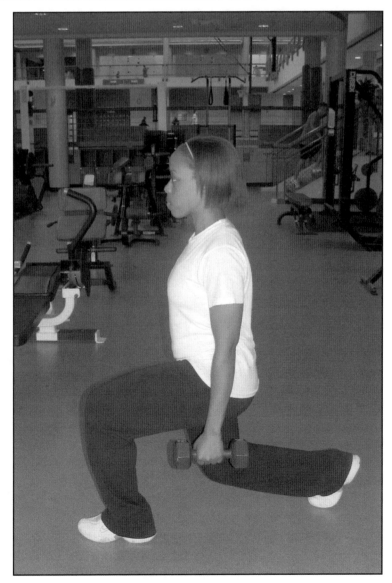

LOWER-BODY EXERCISES

Exercise	Number of Joints and Muscle Groups Involved	Description
Leg Extensions	**Single-joint:** Knee **Primary:** Quadriceps	Sit on the machine and line the middle of your knee up with the mechanical pivot point of the machine. You may accomplish this by sliding the back rest forward or backward accordingly. The leg adjustment should be between your ankles and lower portion of your calf muscle. Keeping your hips against the back rest and while holding onto the handles, extend your lower leg until it is fully extended and then return to the starting position (just before the weight stack touches). Repeat until you have completed the desired number of repetitions.

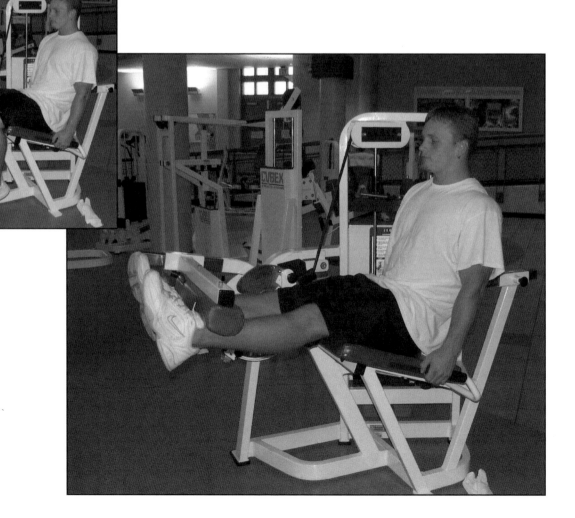

LOWER-BODY EXERCISES

Exercise	Number of Joints and Muscle Groups Involved	Description
Seated Leg Curls	**Single-joint:** Knee **Primary:** Hamstrings	Sit on the machine and line the middle of your knee up with the mechanical pivot point of the machine. You may accomplish this by sliding the back rest forward or backward accordingly. Using the handle on the right side, push the handle forward, lowering the leg rest and place your legs in the leg rest. Keeping your hips against the back rest and while holding onto the handles, flex your lower leg until it is at roughly 90 degrees and then return to the starting position (just before the machine hits the stopper). Repeat until you have completed the desired number of repetitions.

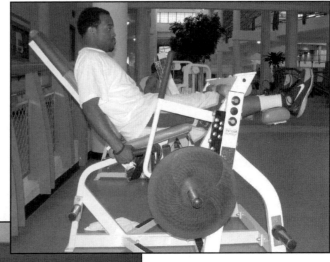

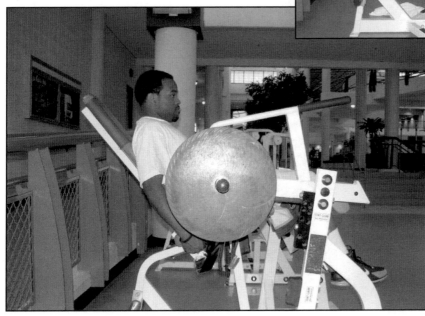

LOWER-BODY EXERCISES

Exercise	Number of Joints and Muscle Groups Involved	Description
Prone Leg Curls	**Single-joint:** Knee **Primary:** Hamstrings	In the prone position, line your knees up with the mechanical pivot point of the machine. Adjust the leg rest so that it will lie between your calf and ankle. While grasping the handles and keeping your head in a neutral position, flex your knees by pulling your heels toward your buttocks. Do not allow your hips or thighs to lift off of the bench. Slowly lower your heels back to the starting position (just before the weight stack touches). Repeat until you have completed the desired number of repetitions.

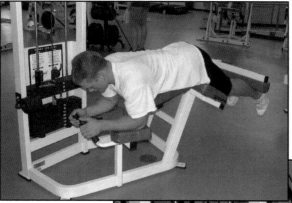

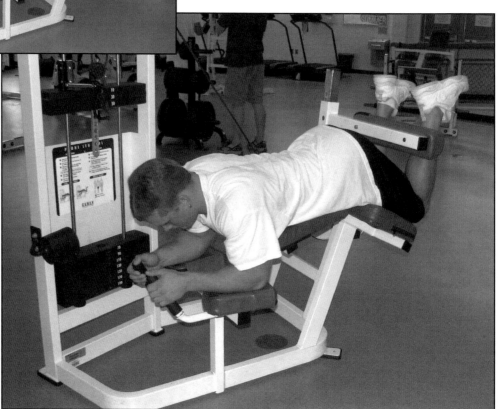

LOWER-BODY EXERCISES

Exercise	Number of Joints and Muscle Groups Involved	Description
Standing Calf Raises	**Multi-joint:** Ankle and Ball of foot **Primary:** Gastrocnemius	Standing on the foot rest facing the weight stack, position your feet with the balls of your feet on the top, allowing your heels to hang off. Place your shoulder under the shoulder pads; you may have to adjust the pad by pulling the pin and raising or lowering the pad accordingly. Keeping your back straight and toes pointing straight ahead, push up on your toes, raising your heels as high as possible. Slowly lower your heels to the start position and repeat until desired repetitions are completed.

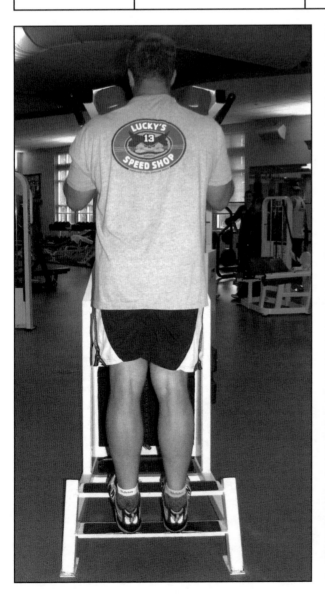
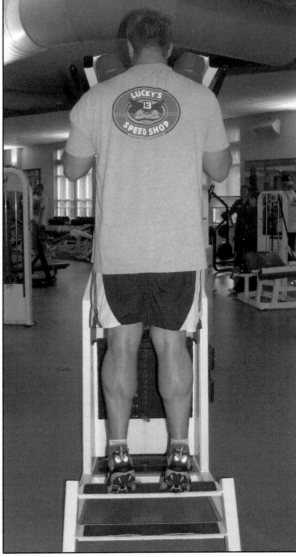

LOWER-BODY EXERCISES

Exercise	Number of Joints and Muscle Groups Involved	Description
Hip Adductors	**Single-joint:** Hips **Primary:** Hip Adductors	Sit on the machine placing your feet in the foot rest and your knees in contact with the pads. Pull the handle on your right side and spread your feet apart until you feel a good stretch in your groin. Bring your knees together by pressing inward on the knee pads. Slowly return to the starting position (just before the weight stack touches). Repeat until desired number of repetitions are complete. Afterward, pull the hand to your right and return your legs to the initial position.

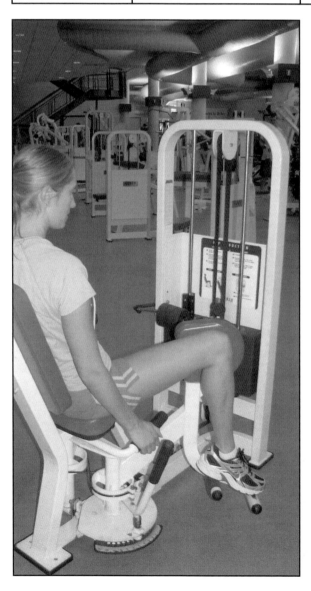
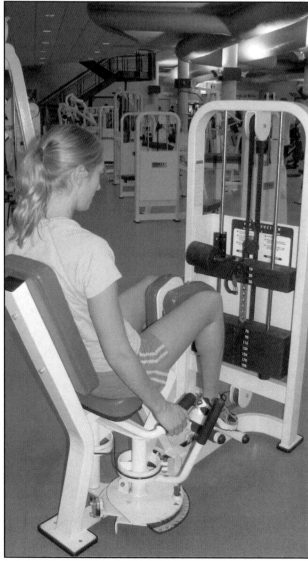

LOWER-BODY EXERCISES

Exercise	Number of Joints and Muscle Groups Involved	Description
Hip Abductors	**Single-joint:** Hips **Primary:** Hip Abuctors	Sit on the machine placing your feet in the foot rest and your knees in contact with the pads. Pull the handle on your right side and bring your legs together. Spread your knees apart by pressing outward on the knee pads. Slowly return to the starting position (just before the weight stack touches). Repeat until the desired number of repetitions are complete. Afterwards, pull the hand to your right and return your legs to the initial position.

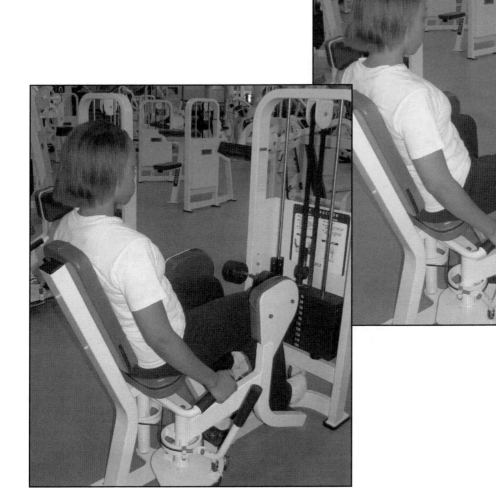

UPPER-BODY EXERCISES

Exercise	Number of Joints and Muscle Groups Involved	Description
Barbell Bench Press	**Multi-joint:** Shoulder and Elbow **Primary:** Pectoralis Major **Secondary:** Anterior Deltoid and Triceps	Start off by lying on your back on a flat bench with your head and buttocks in contact with the bench and feet flat on the floor. Keep your back in a natural alignment (this will vary from person to person). Grasp the barbell with an overhand grip slightly wider than shoulder width. After un-racking the barbell, slowly lower the bar to the lower portion of your chest (right below your nipples) in a controlled motion. Immediately afterwards, push the bar upwards avoiding bouncing the bar off your chest or lifting your buttocks off the bench. Repeat until you have completed the desired number of repetitions.

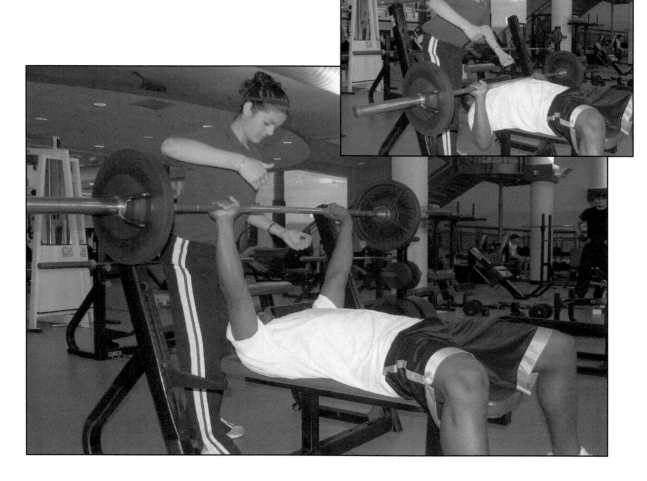

UPPER-BODY EXERCISES

Exercise	Number of Joints and Muscle Groups Involved	Description
Dumbell Incline Press	**Multi-joint:** Shoulder and Elbow **Primary:** Pectoralis Major **Secondary:** Anterior Deltoid and Triceps	Start off by laying on your back on an incline bench with your head and buttocks in contact with the bench and feet flat on the floor. Keep your back in a natural alignment (this will vary from person to person). Hold the dumbbells by your shoulders with palms of your hands facing away from your body. Keeping the dumbbells over your chest, slowly extend your shoulders and elbows upwards and bring your hands together. Slowly return the dumbbells to the starting position and repeat until desired number of repetitions are complete.

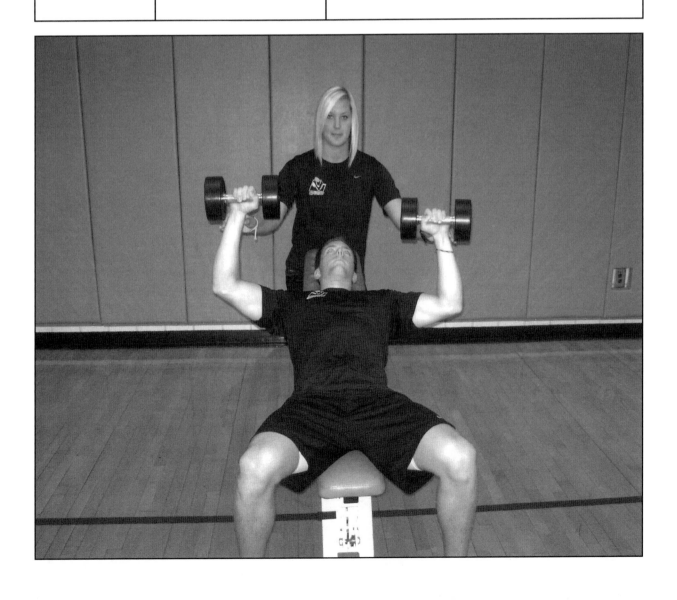

UPPER-BODY EXERCISES

Exercise	Number of Joints and Muscle Groups Involved	Description

Pull Downs	**Multi-joint:**
	    Shoulder and Elbow
	
	Primary:
	    Latissimus Dorsi,
	    Trapezius, Rhomboid,
	    and Posterior Deltoid
	Secondary:
	    Biceps
		Before sitting down, assume an overhand or under-hand grip roughly shoulder width apart. Sit facing the machine with your thighs under the padding above your knee. You may have to adjust the knee pad by pulling the pin and raising or lowering the pad accordingly. Once in position, slightly lean back and pull the bar down to the top portion of your sternum and slowly allow the bar to return to the starting position. Repeat until you have completed the desired number of repetitions.

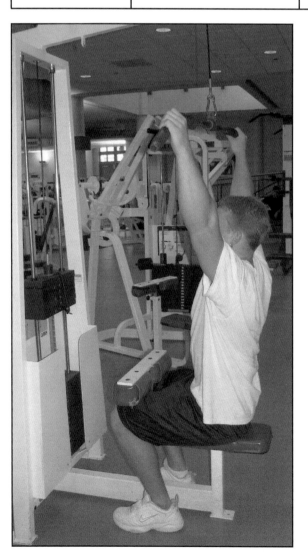
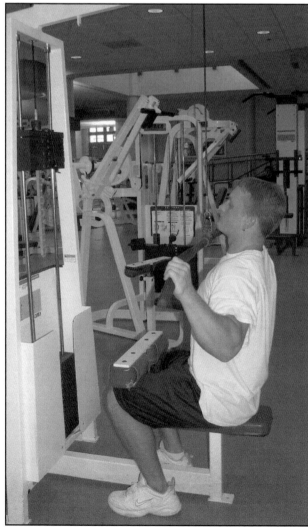

UPPER-BODY EXERCISES

Exercise	Number of Joints and Muscle Groups Involved	Description

Assisted Pull-ups	**Multi-joint:**
	    Shoulder and Elbow
	
	Primary:
	    Latissimus Dorsi, Trapezius, Rhomboid, and Posterior Deltoid
	Secondary:
	    Biceps
		Stand on the second step (first step for taller individuals) and grasp the overhead bars. Step onto the foot rest and lower your body until your arms are fully extended over your head. Slowly pull yourself up until your hands are by your shoulders and elbows by your side. Return to the beginning position and repeat until desired repetitions are complete. ***NOTE:*** The more weight you use on this machine the easier the movement will become.

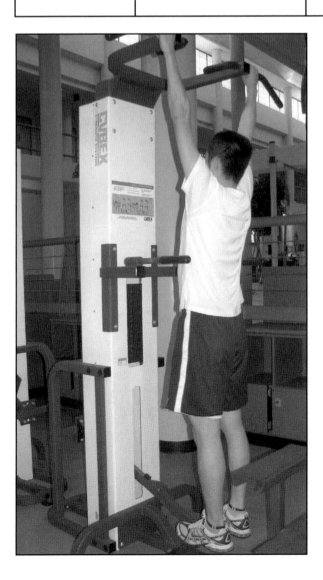

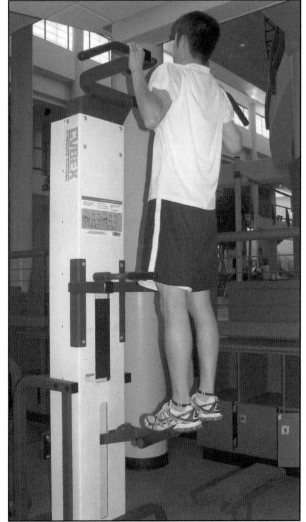

UPPER-BODY EXERCISES

Exercise	Number of Joints and Muscle Groups Involved	Description

Seated Low Row	**Multi-joint:**
	    Shoulder and Elbow
	
	Primary:
	    Latissimus Dorsi, Trapezius, Rhomboid, and Posterior Deltoid
	Secondary:
	    Biceps
		Sit in an upright position facing the handles with your feet resting on the floor. Slightly lean forward and grab the handles with both hands, keeping your chest in contact with the pad. Keeping your elbows by your side, pull the handle to the lower portion of your chest/upper abdominal region, squeezing your shoulder blades together in the process. Slowly return the weight to the starting position. Repeat until you have completed the desired number of repetitions.

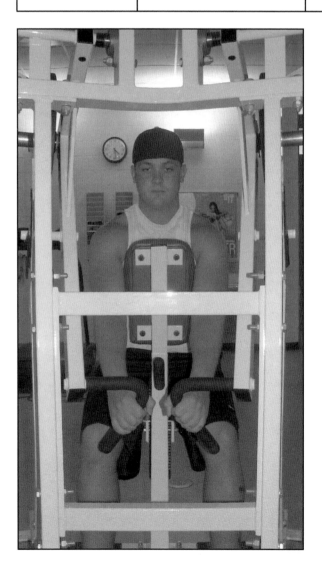

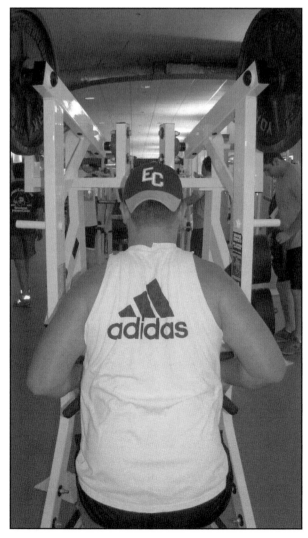

UPPER-BODY EXERCISES

Exercise	Number of Joints and Muscle Groups Involved	Description
Machine Overhead Press	**Single-joint:** Shoulder and Elbow **Primary:** Anterior and Medial Head of Deltoid **Secondary:** Triceps	Before sitting down, adjust seat so that the handles are just above shoulder height. Begin the exercise with elbows flexed at 90 degrees. In a smooth, controlled manner, extend your arms overhead but do not lock out your elbows. Then lower your arms back to the starting position. Repeat until you have completed the desired number of repetitions.

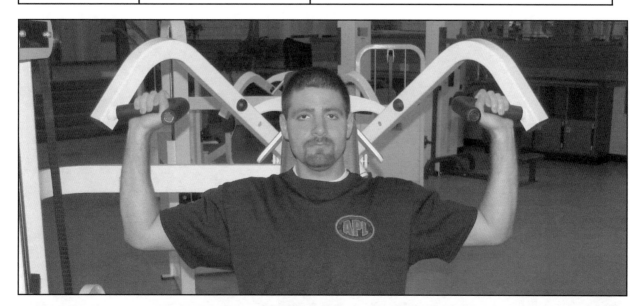

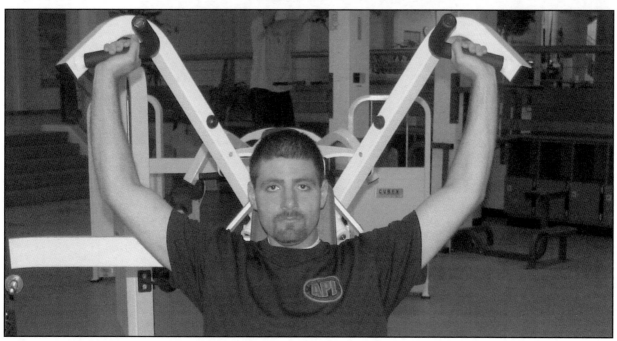

UPPER-BODY EXERCISES

Exercise	Number of Joints and Muscle Groups Involved	Description
Lateral Dumbell Raises	**Single-joint:** Shoulder **Primary:** Medial Head of Deltoid	Stand or sit with a straight back holding two dumbbells by your side. Your arms should be slightly flexed but in a fixed position. Laterally raise your arms until dumbbells are parallel to the floor and then lower them to your sides. Repeat until you have completed the desired number of repetitions.

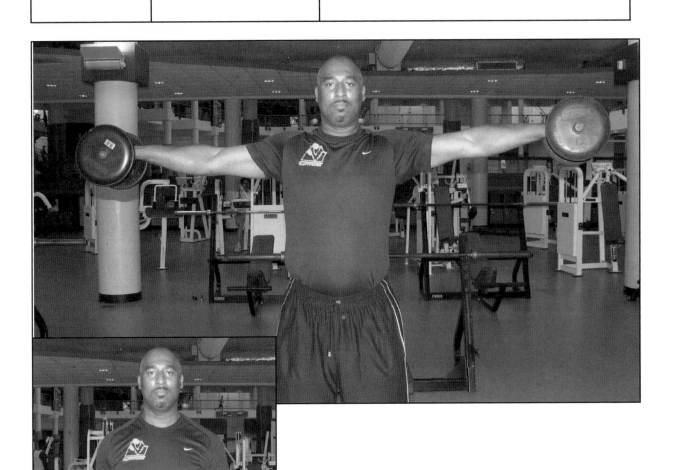

UPPER-BODY EXERCISES

Exercise	Number of Joints and Muscle Groups Involved	Description
Machine Arm Curls	**Single-joint:** Elbow **Primary:** Biceps	Sit on the machine with your torso over the arm padding and line the middle of your elbow up with the mechanical pivot point of the machine. You may accomplish this by sliding the seat up and down accordingly. With an underhand grip keeping your arms parallel to one another, slowly flex your lower arm pulling the handle upward, keeping your upper arms in contact with the arm pad the entire time. Then return the handle to the starting position (just before the weight stack touches). Repeat until you have completed the desired number of repetitions.

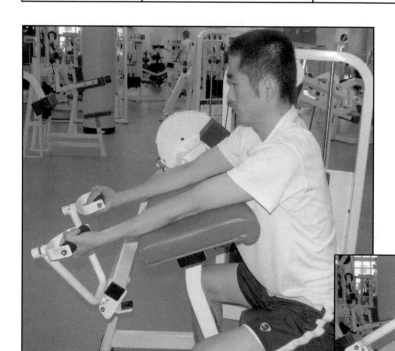

UPPER-BODY EXERCISES

Exercise	Number of Joints and Muscle Groups Involved	Description
Hammer Curls	**Single-joint:** Elbow **Primary:** Biceps	Stand upright with dumbbells in both hands. Holding each dumbbell with a neutral grip (palms facing your body) and keeping your elbow by your side, slowly flex your arm bringing the dumbbell by your shoulder. Return the dumbbell to the starting position and repeat on the other side.

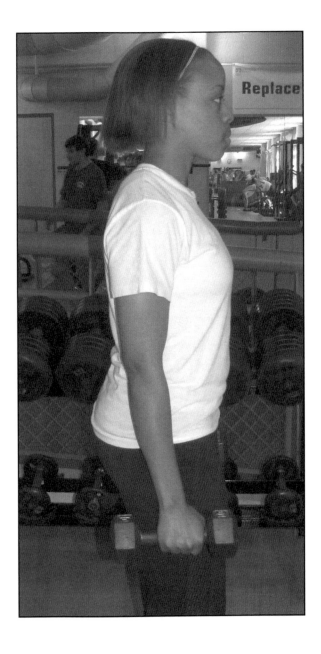
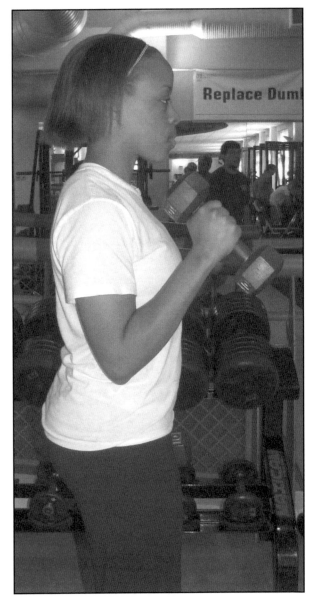

UPPER-BODY EXERCISES

Exercise	Number of Joints and Muscle Groups Involved	Description
Assisted Dip	**Multi-joint:** Shoulder and Elbow **Primary:** Pectoralis Major, Anterior Deltoid, and Triceps	Stand on the second step (first for taller individuals) and grasp the parallel bars. Step onto the foot rest and extend your arms so that your torso is over the bars. With your legs and trunk extended the entire time, slowly lower your body until your elbows are flexed 90 degrees. Then extend your arm back to the beginning position and repeat until you have completed the desired number of repetitions. NOTE: The more weight you use on this machine the easier the movement will become.

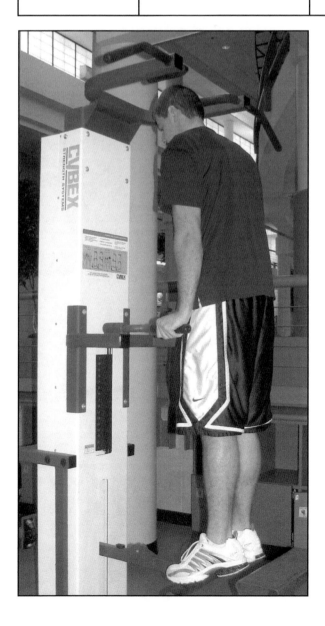
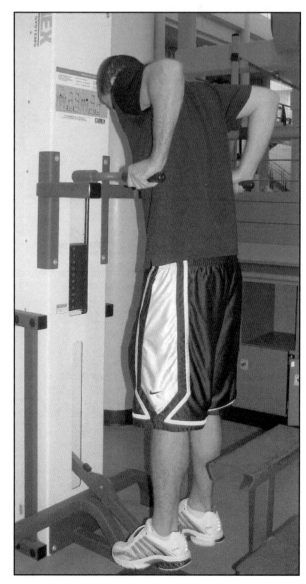

UPPER-BODY EXERCISES

Exercise	Number of Joints and Muscle Groups Involved	Description
Press Downs	**Single-joint:** Elbow **Primary:** Triceps	Grab the bar with a shoulder width grip keeping your elbows by your side. Standing straight with your knees slightly flexed, extend your arms down toward your waist. Again keeping your elbows by your side, slowly flex the arms back to the starting position and repeat until you have completed the desired number of repetitions.

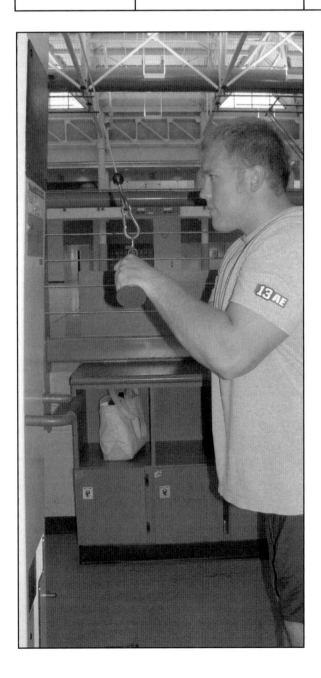 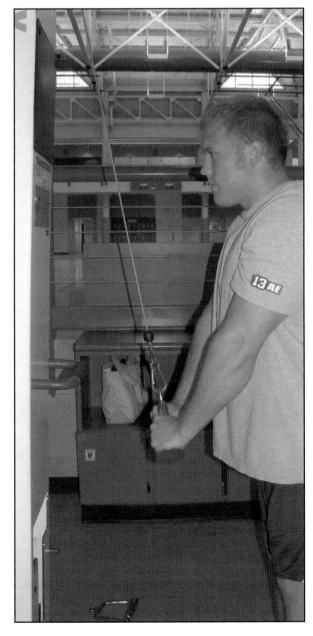

UPPER-BODY EXERCISES

Exercise	Number of Joints and Muscle Groups Involved	Description
Machine Arm Extensions	**Single-joint:** Elbow **Primary:** Triceps	Sit on the machine with your torso over the arm padding and line the middle of your elbow up with the mechanical pivot point of the machine. You may accomplish this by sliding the seat up and down accordingly. In order to keep your torso in contact with the arm pad, you may move the back rest accordingly. With a neutral grip, keeping your arms parallel to one another, slowly extend your lower arm while pushing the handle away from your body and keeping your upper arms in contact with the arm pad the entire time. Then return the handle to the starting position (just before the weight stack touches). Repeat until you have completed the desired number of repetitions.

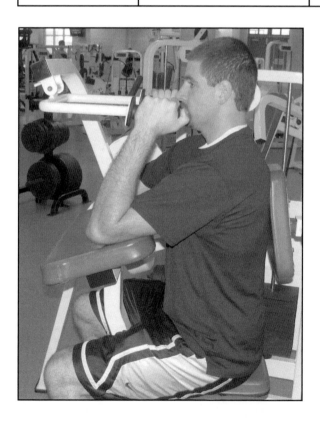 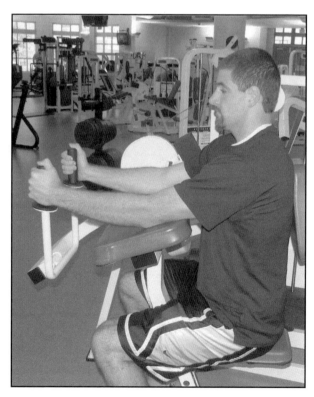

CORE EXERCISES

Exercise	Number of Joints and Muscle Groups Involved	Description
Crunch	**Single-joint:** Vertebral Column **Primary:** Rectus Abdominis	Lie on your back with your arms across your chest. You may also place both hands behind your head to support the weight of your head, but remember never pull on your head. Legs should be bent with your feet flat on the floor. Keeping your head in a neutral position, slowly raise your shoulder blades off the floor. Think about pulling your sternum down towards your pelvis. Slowly lower your shoulder blades back to the floor and repeat until desired repetitions are complete.

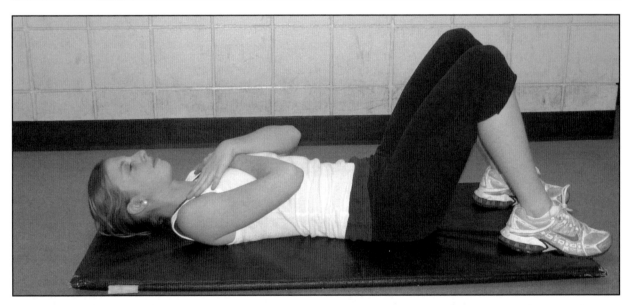

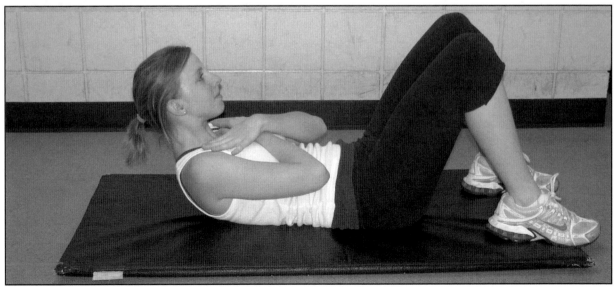

CORE EXERCISES

Exercise	Number of Joints and Muscle Groups Involved	Description

Stability Crunch	**Single-joint:**
	   Vertebral Column
	
	Primary:
	   Rectus Abdominis
		Lie on your back with your arms across your chest. You may also place both hands behind your head to support the weight of your head, but remember never pull on your head. Legs should be bent with your feet flat on the floor. Keeping your head in a neutral position, slowly raise your shoulder blades off the floor. Think about pulling your sternum down towards your pelvis. Slowly lower your shoulder blades back to the floor and repeat until desired repetitions are complete.

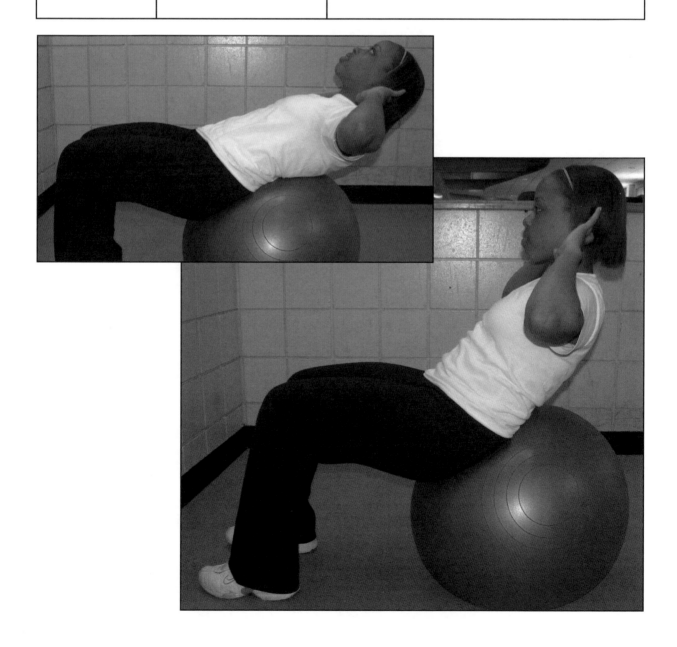

CORE EXERCISES

Exercise	Number of Joints and Muscle Groups Involved	Description
Reverse Crunch	**Multi-joint:** Vertebral Column **Primary:** Rectus Abdominis and Hip Flexors	With your hands under your buttocks to flatten your lower back. Elevate your feet with your knees bent at 90 degrees and directly over your hips. Using the lower portion of your abdominal wall, raise your hips off of your hands or the floor three to six inches. Now slowly lower your hips back to your hands or the floor and repeat until desired number of repetitions are complete.

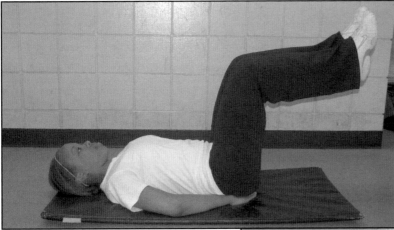

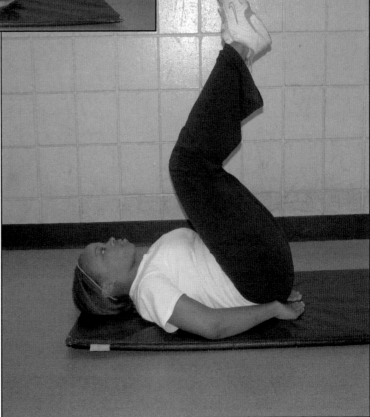

CORE EXERCISES

Exercise	Number of Joints and Muscle Groups Involved	Description
Hanging Knee Raises	**Multi-joint:** Hips and Vertebral Column **Primary:** Rectus Abdominis and Hip Flexors	Support your body by resting your elbows and lower arms on the arm pads and grasp handles. With your legs hanging, position your back against the back support and raise your knees towards your chest. Slowly lower your legs back to the beginning position and repeat until desired repetitions are complete.

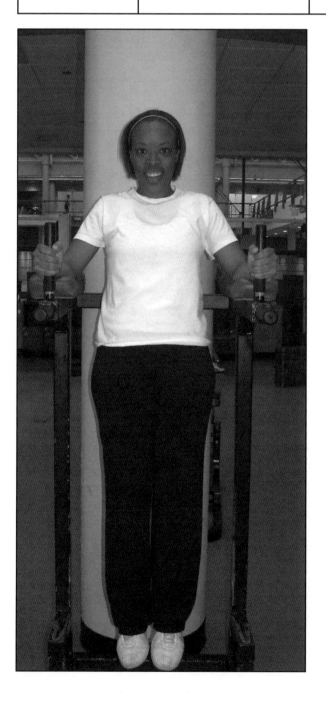
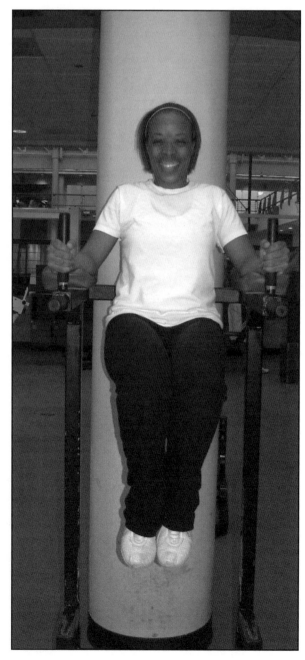

CORE EXERCISES

Exercise	Number of Joints and Muscle Groups Involved	Description
Stability Ball Jacknife	**Multi-joint:** Hips and Vertebral Column **Primary:** Rectus Abdominis and Hip Flexors	Squat down behind and put your abdomen on top of the stability ball. Now roll forward so that your hands reach the ground in front of the ball. Walk out until your feet are on top of the ball. Hold this push-up position keeping a strong core. Bend your knees and pull the ball up toward your chest. Extend your legs to move the ball to where you began and repeat until desired repetitions are complete.

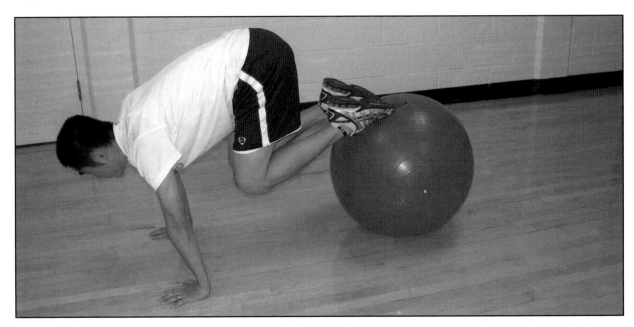

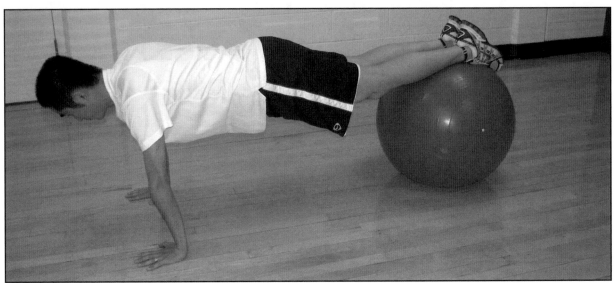

CORE EXERCISES

Exercise	Number of Joints and Muscle Groups Involved	Description
Machine Back Extensions	**Single-joint:** Hip **Primary:** Erector Spinae	Sit on the machine with the upper portion of your back against the back rest. Adjust the foot plate so that your hips are in line with the mechanical pivot point of the machine. Your feet should be flat on the foot plate with a slight bend in your knees. Crossing your arms over your chest, extend your torso until you are fully extended but not hyperextended. Slowly allow your torso to flex forward toward the starting position (just before the weight stack touches). Repeat until the desired number of repetitions are complete.

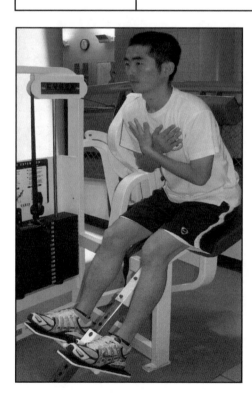

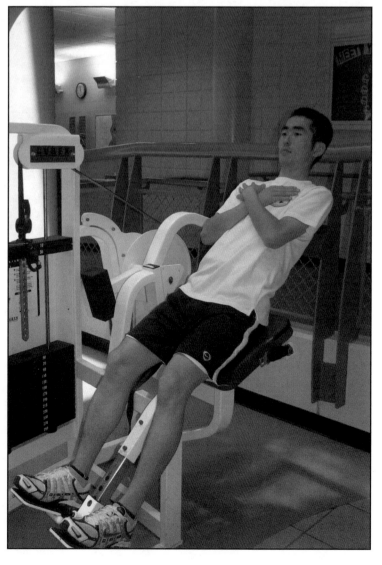

CORE EXERCISES

Exercise	Number of Joints and Muscle Groups Involved	Description

Trunk Lift	**Single-joint:**
	    Vertebral Column
	
	Primary:
	    Erector Spinae
		Lie face down on the floor with your arms by your side. Keeping your head straight slowly raise your shoulders and chest off the floor and hold for one second. Slowly return to beginning position and repeat until desire repetitions are complete.

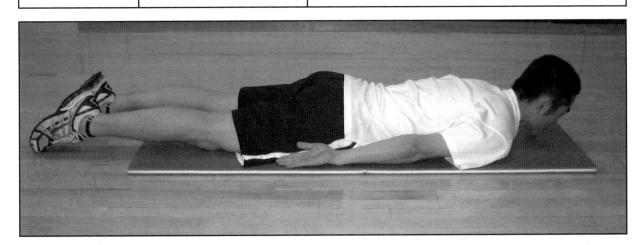

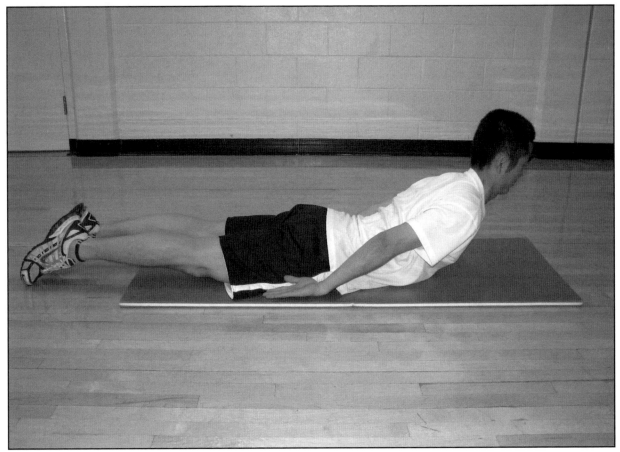

CORE EXERCISES

Exercise	Number of Joints and Muscle Groups Involved	Description
Prone Plank	**Primary:** Core Stabilizers	Lie face down on the floor resting your forearms and elbows on the floor. Keeping your core tight, elevate your body so that only your toes, elbows, and forearms are on the floor. Hold for 10 to 30 seconds and repeat. Alternative: Place hands on floor like push-up.

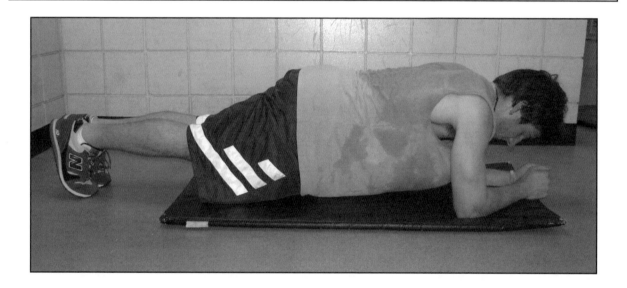

Side Plank	**Primary:** Core Stabilizers	Lie on your side placing the elbow closest to the floor on the floor. Slowly raise your body up keeping only your foot, elbow, and forearm (same side of body) in contact with the floor. Hold position for 10 to 30 seconds and repeat.

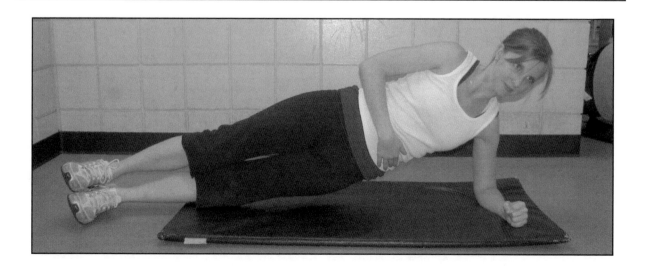

CORE EXERCISES

Exercise	Number of Joints and Muscle Groups Involved	Description
Stability Ball Balance	**Primary:** Core Stabilizers	Place both knees on the ball while keeping both hands in contact with the floor. One at a time, take one hand off the floor and place it on the stability ball. Again take one hand off the ball and hold it to your side and balance. Try to hold this position for 10 to 30 seconds and relax.

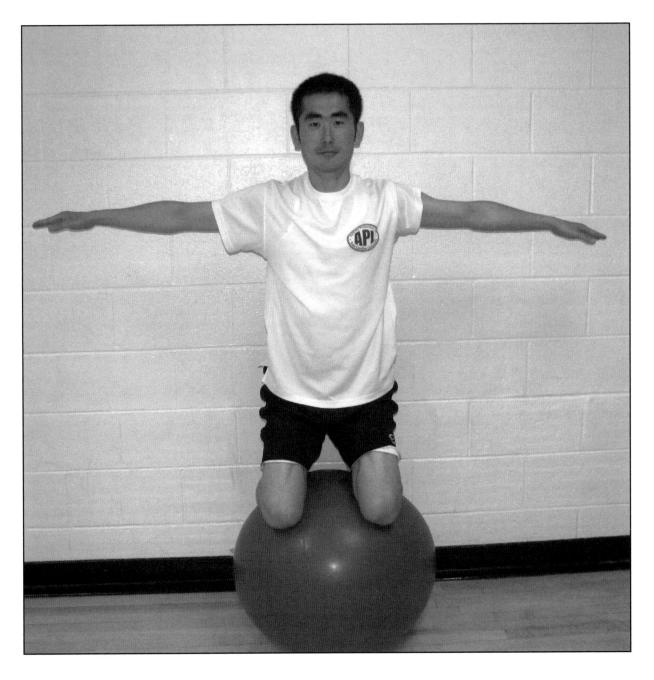

APPENDIX FIVE

SAMPLE TRAINING PROGRAMS

LOWER-BODY STRENGTH WORKOUT

Exercise	Set 1 Reps	Set 2 Reps	Set 3 Reps	Set 4 Reps
Back squat	70% 1-RM x 6 reps	70% 1-RM x 6 reps	0% 1-RM x 6 reps	70% 1-RM x 6 reps
Lunges	6 reps each leg	6 reps each leg	6 reps each leg	6 reps each leg
Leg press	8 reps	8 reps	8 reps	
Leg curl	10 reps	10 reps	10 reps	
Seated calf raises	10 reps	10 reps	10 reps	

UPPER-BODY STRENGTH WORKOUT

Exercise	Set 1 Reps	Set 2 Reps	Set 3 Reps	Set 4 Reps
Barbell bench press	70% 1-RM x 6 reps	70% 1-RM x 6 reps	70% 1-RM x 6 reps	70% 1-RM x 6 reps
Bent-over row	6 reps	6 reps	6 reps	6 reps
Dumbbell shoulder press	8 reps	8 reps	8 reps	8 reps
Pull-downs	8 reps	8 reps	8 reps	
Dips	10 reps	10 reps	10 reps	
Hammer curls	10 reps	10 reps	10 reps	

LOWER-BODY HYPERTROPHY WORKOUT

Exercise	Set 1 Reps	Set 2 Reps	Set 3 Reps	Set 4 Reps	Set 5 Reps
Back Squat	60% 1-RM x 8 reps	60% 1-RM x 8 reps	60% 1-RM x 8 reps	60% 1-RM x 8 reps	60% 1-RM x 8 reps
Lunges	8 reps each leg	8 reps each leg	8 reps each leg	8 reps each leg	8 reps each leg
Prone leg curls	12 reps	12 reps	12 reps		
Leg extensions	12 reps	12 reps	12 reps		
Standing calf raises	15 reps	15 reps	15 reps		

UPPER-BODY HYPERTROPHY WORKOUT

Exercise	Set 1 Reps	Set 2 Reps	Set 3 Reps	Set 4 Reps	Set 5 Reps
Barbell bench press	60% 1-RM x 8 reps	60% 1-RM x 8 reps	60% 1-RM x 8 reps	60% 1-RM x 8 reps	60% 1-RM x 8 reps
Bent-over row	8 reps	8 reps	8 reps	8 reps	8 reps
Dumbbell shoulder press	10 reps	10 reps	10 reps		
Pull-downs	10 reps	10 reps	10 reps		
Lateral dumbbell raises	12 reps	12 reps	12 reps		
Hammer curls	12 reps	12 reps	12 reps		
Press-downs	12 reps	12 reps	12 reps		

LOWER-BODY MUSCULAR ENDURANCE WORKOUT

Exercise	Set 1 Reps	Set 2 Reps	Set 3 Reps
Back Squat	50% 1-RM x 12 reps	50% 1-RM x 12 reps	50% 1-RM x 12 reps
Lunges	12 reps	12 reps	12 reps
Leg extensions	15 reps	15 reps	15 reps
Prone leg curls	15 reps	15 reps	15 reps
Hip adduction	15 reps	15 reps	15 reps
Seated calf raises	20 reps	20 reps	

UPPER-BODY MUSCULAR ENDURANCE WORKOUT

Exercise	Set 1 Reps	Set 2 Reps	Set 3 Reps
Barbell bench press	50% 1-RM x 12 reps	50% 1-RM x 12 reps	50% 1-RM x 12 reps
Seated low row	15 reps	15 reps	15 reps
Lateral dumbbell raises	15 reps	15 reps	15 reps
Assisted dips	15 reps	15 reps	15 reps
Press-downs	15 reps	15 reps	15 reps
Machine arm curls	20 reps	20 reps	

TOTAL-BODY PLYOMETRIC WORKOUT

Exercise	Set 1 Reps	Set 2 Reps	Set 3 Reps
Squat jumps	6 reps	6 reps	6 reps
Med ball pass	6 reps	6 reps	6 reps
Ice skaters	6 reps each leg	6 reps each leg	6 reps each leg
Med ball overhead toss	6 reps	6 reps	6 reps

BODYWEIGHT CIRCUIT TRAINING

Exercise	20–30 sec (Reps)	Rounds
Squats	AMAP	3 – 5
Push-ups	AMAP	
Jump rope	AMAP	
Mountain climber	AMAP	
Crunches	AMAP	

CORE WORKOUT

Exercise	Set 1 Reps or Sec	Set 2 Reps or Sec	Set 3 Reps or Sec
Prone plank	30 – 60 sec.	30 – 60 sec.	30 – 60 sec.
Crunch	15 – 30 reps	15 – 30 reps	15 – 30 reps
Hanging knee raises	15 – 30 reps	15 – 30 reps	15 – 30 reps
Trunk lift	15 – 30 reps	15 – 30 reps	15 – 30 reps
Side plank	20 – 30 sec.	20 – 30 sec.	20 – 30 sec.

APPENDIX SIX

FLEXIBILITY AND STRETCHING

LOWER-BODY STRETCHES

Exercise and Muscle Group Stretched	Description
Modified Hurdler: Hamstrings	While sitting on the floor, extend one leg out and bring the opposite foot near the side of the knee that is extended. Keeping the extended leg straight, slowly flex the spine and hips and reach for your foot. If you cannot grab your foot, reach for your ankle or calf instead. Hold stretch and repeat on the other side.

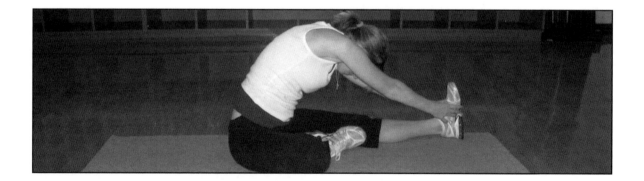

LOWER-BODY STRETCHES

Exercise and Muscle Group Stretched	Description
Standing Toe Hold: Quadriceps	Stand up straight with feet shoulder width apart and toes pointing straight ahead. Flex one leg bringing your heel towards your buttocks and hold with the hand on the same side. In order to help you keep your balance, locate a fixed object and keep your eyes on that object. Hold stretch and repeat on the other side.

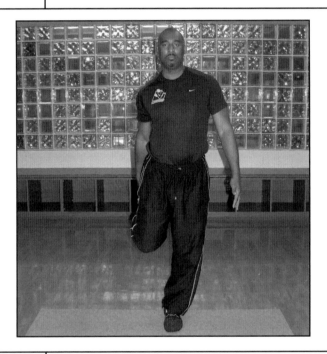

Exercise and Muscle Group Stretched	Description
Forward Lunge: Quadriceps and Hip Flexors	Stand with feet shoulder width apart and take one step forward. In this position, slightly bend both knees and tilt your pelvis forward by shifting your hips under your shoulders. Hold stretch and repeat on other side.

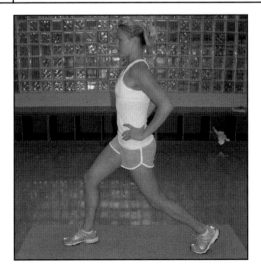

LOWER-BODY STRETCHES

Exercise and Muscle Group Stretched	Description
Wall Stretch: Gastrocnemius	Find a wall or immovable object and place both hands on the wall above shoulder height. Place one leg behind the other and shift your weight forward. In the process, keep the back heel in contact with the floor.

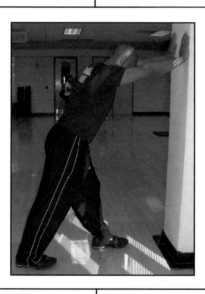 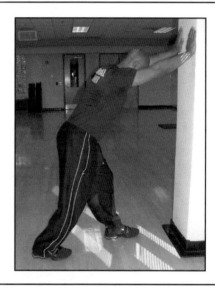

Exercise and Muscle Group Stretched	Description
Butterfly: Hip Flexors and Adductors	Sit down on the floor and place the bottom of each foot together and pull your heels in towards the body. Keeping your chest up, grasp each ankle and place your elbows inside of your knees. While pulling your ankles in, slightly apply downward pressure on each knee and hold stretch.

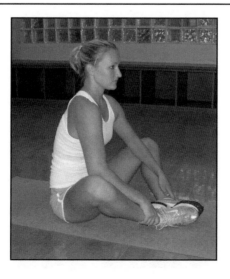

UPPER-BODY STRETCHES

Exercise and Muscle Group Stretched	Description

Hands Behind Back: Pectoralis Major	Standing with feet shoulder width apart, place both arms behind your back and grasp hands together. Slowly raise both arms keeping your elbows straight and head and neck relaxed. Hold stretch and repeat.

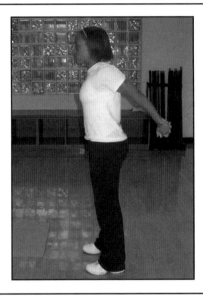

Behind the Neck: Triceps and Latissimus Dorsi	Standing with feet shoulder width apart, raise one arm while flexing that same elbow. Using your opposite arm, reach for your elbow. Slightly pull down and inward. Hold stretch and repeat on the other side.

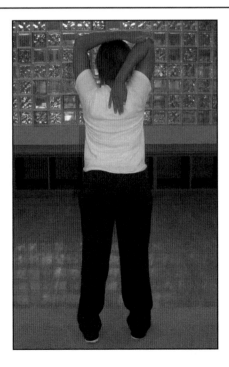

UPPER-BODY STRETCHES

Exercise and Muscle Group Stretched	Description

| **Neck Stretch:** Sternocleidomastoid, Suboccipitals, and Splenae | Standing with your feet should width apart, slowly turn your head to one side. Hold stretch and repeat on the other side. Next flex your neck bringing your chin toward your sternum and hold. Then hyperextend your neck and try to touch your head to your upper back and hold. |

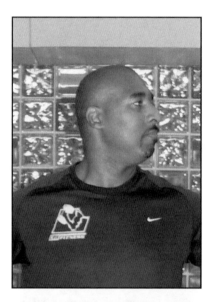
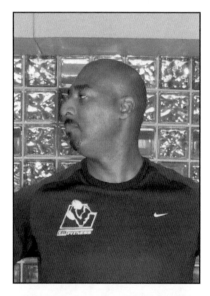
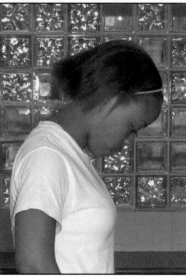
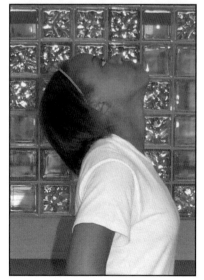

THERE'S AN APP FOR THAT

MYWELLNESS CLOUD

This is a free app that allows you to track all daily movement including physical activity, exercise and daily functional movement done inside of a recreation center, at home, or outdoors. Daily MOVE goals are set for you based on your recent activity level; the goals adapt as your fitness adapts. In addition, this app allows you to connect other devices and accounts to make tracking activity simple and concise. Accounts you can link to the MyWellness cloud include:

- Fit Bit
- Garmin
- Map My Fitness
- My Fitness Pal
- Polar
- Run Keeper
- Strava
- Swimtag
- Withings

WALKJOGRUN

This app provides pace coaching, which allows you to pick a pace for your workout or race and the pace coach will tell you when to speed up or when to slow down in order to meet your goal!

SWORK IT

The free app is built to work around anyone's schedule and is great if time is a factor in your fitness, workouts in as little as 5 minutes if needed. The workouts require no equipment and you can select from 20 pre-built workouts or create your own that focuses on cardio, strength, yoga or flexibility. Video instruction and audio cues are provided to take you through the workout and make it easy to follow along.

POPSUGAR ACTIVE

Create and customize workout routines from the videos made available through this app. It also provides preloaded workouts. Workouts include yoga, HIIT, Tabata, strength training, and core training.

MAPMYRUN

This app is free. It allows you to map your runs using a GPS and set up a personal profile. In addition, this app allows you to:

- Find running routes others have completed near your current location.

- Log your workouts.
- Log daily nutrition information and keep up with your caloric intake.
- Interact with others via various social media such as Facebook and Twitter.

MYFITNESSPAL

This free app includes a food database to choose items you have eaten. In addition, this app allows you to:

- Keep track of everything you eat—a food diary and all of your exercise activity.
- Show your daily caloric intake and caloric expenditure.
- Scan bar codes on various food items to log the item into your diary.
- Make goals.

LIVEHAPPY

Psychology in a simple form for everyday use. This app is based on scientific research and contains motivational ways to stay positive. It allows you to incorporate short-term and long-term goal setting for any life situation while evaluating your extrinsic and intrinsic motivations.

PUMPING WEIGHT

An ideal app for tracking workout routines with a smooth and straightforward workout log. It provides illustrations and instructions for more than 200 exercises! It also includes an interval timer and a rest timer.

FOODUCATE

This app allows you to really see the quality of the food you choose. Simply scan the barcode of the food item to see what's really in it. But Fooducate won't leave you hanging; it will also provide you with a healthier option than the one you've chosen. You can track your food intake along with your exercise.

GYM BOSS 2 INTERVAL TIMER

This is a programmable interval timer ideal for cardio workouts or HIIT training. You can create your own timers specific to your workouts.

INSTANT HEART RATE

Measure your heart rate instantly by placing the tip of your index finger on your smartphone's camera. The app will beep along with your pulse while also providing a real-time chart showing every beat. This app also allows you to store data for up to one week.

YOGAGLO

Yoga routines for everyone. If you are a member, you can choose yoga for women, cyclists, teachers, or beginners. You also have the option to choose a specific yoga instructor, yoga style such as Ashtanga or Hatha, yoga level, and duration between 5 minutes and 120 minutes.

TABATA PRO

This app is easy to use for weight training, kettlebells, running, cycling, or any type of interval training. With three programmable timers, it allows you to customize the time settings, number of cycles, and number of tabatas. Alerts are easy to hear over your music and the flashing screen is a great visual cue.

MYTHOUGHTS+

MyThoughts+ is a great app to change negative self-talk. Every time you turn it on, it greets you with positive and affirming encouragement. You can also personalize your list of comments best suited for you, or create your own custom affirmations!

YOGA STUDIO

This app is available on Google play or through the iPhone App store. Yoga Studio allows you to have 24-hour access to a yoga classes that are provided through visual and audio instruction. The app includes 65 ready-made yoga classes with beginner, intermediate, and advanced options as well as 15 minute, 30 minute or 60 minutes class times. You can choose to focus on strength, balance, flexibility, relaxation, or a combination.

NIKETRAINING CLUB

This is a free app. It allows you to access various types of workouts anytime, anywhere, based on your personal goals. Options include: Get Lean, Get Toned, Get Strong, and Get Focused. In addition, this app allows you to:

- Track personal progress and workout history.
- Earn workout rewards.
- Receive "Bonus Workouts" each month by professional female athletes such as Kara Goucher, Laura Enever, and Shawn Johnson. The workouts include step-by-step instructions and video demonstrations for each drill.